Randa DHAOUI
Saida HIDOURI

Bronchopulmonary malformations in children

Randa DHAOUI
Saida HIDOURI

Bronchopulmonary malformations in children

Diagnostic and therapeutic problems of
adenomatoid cystic malformations of the lungs

ScienciaScripts

Imprint

Any brand names and product names mentioned in this book are subject to trademark, brand or patent protection and are trademarks or registered trademarks of their respective holders. The use of brand names, product names, common names, trade names, product descriptions etc. even without a particular marking in this work is in no way to be construed to mean that such names may be regarded as unrestricted in respect of trademark and brand protection legislation and could thus be used by anyone.

Cover image: www.ingimage.com

This book is a translation from the original published under ISBN 978-620-6-72095-9.

Publisher:
Sciencia Scripts
is a trademark of
Dodo Books Indian Ocean Ltd. and OmniScriptum S.R.L publishing group

120 High Road, East Finchley, London, N2 9ED, United Kingdom
Str. Armeneasca 28/1, office 1, Chisinau MD-2012, Republic of Moldova, Europe
Printed at: see last page
ISBN: 978-620-3-69500-7

ABSTRACT

The congenital cystic adenomatoid malformation (CCAM) of the lung is a rare abnormality. The diagnosis may be discussed with many other broncho- pulmonary malformations and some acquired diseases.

The aim of our work was to discuss some diagnostic and therapeutic problems of CCAM and prevent an unnecessary lobectomy.

A retrospective study of 14 children operated over 20 years. We perform an analysis of personal cases of diagnostic and therapeutic errors.

The preoperative diagnosis was established on clinical and radiological findings. The diagnosis of CCAM was dismissed by histology which found: interstitial emphysema (1 case), pulmonary infarction (3 cases), bronchiectasis (1 case), pulmonary capillary hemangiomatosis (1 case), lung abscess and unclassified lesions (7 cases) and hybrid lesion (1 case). In 1 case, the diagnosis of pulmonary abcess was rejected and CCAM was established.

The diagnosis and the treatment of CCAM must be based on a multidisciplinary collaboration. The working diagnosis on clinic and radiology requires histological confirmation. Some diagnostic problems require confrontation with warned pathologists to avoid unnecessary lobectomy.

KEY WORDS: *Broncho-pulmonary malformation, congenital cystic adenomatoïd malformation, lung, infant, diagnostic and therapeutic problems, radiology, histopathology, treatment, surgery*

TABLE OF CONTENTS

INTRODUCTION

Adenomatoid cystic malformations of the lung (ACML) are the most common congenital lung malformations [1]. They occur in 1 in 35,000 to 1 in 25,000 pregnancies [2]. They are characterised by abnormal development of the terminal respiratory structures during foetal life, leading to adenomatoid proliferation of bronchiolar elements and cyst formation [3]. MAKP share common features with other congenital lung malformations. Phenotypic overlap strongly suggests pathophysiological mechanisms common to these malformations with different names [2]. MAKP is most often unilateral and focal, confined to one lung lobe. They have been described in both the right and left lobes and seem to predominate in the lower lobes [2]. Early antenatal diagnosis enables neonatal management [4, 5]. This malformation is most often diagnosed in the perinatal period, but in some cases it can be detected during childhood and adolescence [6]. The clinical picture is variable and sometimes misleading, which may lead to over- or under-diagnosis and treatment errors [7]. Diagnosis is anatomopathological.

The aim of this work is to:

▶ To report a personal series o f diagnostic and therapeutic errors in patients operated on with a diagnosis of excess or defective MAKP, reviewing cases in the literature.

▶ Discuss the diagnostic and therapeutic problems of MAKP that may arise with certain congenital or acquired conditions.

▶ Insist on multidisciplinary collaboration to develop a strategy the most appropriate treatment for certain bronchopulmonary malformations in order t o prevent unnecessary removal.

In this work, we are not talking about "our exploits" but rather about "our mistakes" and trying to learn "lessons" from them, a s literature does not seem to report such series.

CHAPTER I
PATIENTS AND METHODS

This is a retrospective study of 14 observations, carried out in the Paediatric Surgery Department of the Fattouma Bourguiba University Hospital in Monastir, over a 20-year period from January 1993 to December 2012. During the same period, 47 patients underwent surgery for MAKP confirmed by anatomopathology. An antenatal diagnosis was possible in 4 cases. Patients were referred by the Sfax Neonatology Department and the Monastir, Mahdia and Kairouan Paediatrics Departments. Data were collected from medical records and radiological, operative and anatomopathological reports.

1. Inclusion criteria

The criteria included in this work related to:
• Patients operated on with a strong preoperative suspicion of MAKP and in whom anatomopathology has not revealed signs in favour of this condition.
• Patients operated on for another pathology, such as a lung abscess, and in whom anatomopathology confirmed the diagnosis of MAKP. In this group (only one case), a partial resection of the lung tissue was carried out (and not a lobectomy), leaving MAKP tissue in situ.

2. Parameters studied

We have defined the above 9 parameters for our study.

1. The age of onset of symptoms.
2. The age of diagnosis, which generally corresponds to the age of treatment surgical.
3. Clinical symptoms.
4. Associated malformations.
5. Data from imaging and other investigations.
6. Treatment methods.
7. The hospital stay.
8. Clinical and radiological evolution in the medium and long term.
9. Pathological findings.

All patients underwent standard chest X-ray and computed tomography (CT). Thoracic Doppler ultrasonography was performed in 2 cases, oeso-gastro-duodenal transit (TOGD) in 4

4

cases, pulmonary perfusion scintigraphy and respiratory endoscopic exploration in 1 case each.Follow-up was based on clinical and radiological examinations at the outpatient clinic.

Our patients can be classified into 2 groups on the basis of radiological findings:

- Multicystic aortic lesion affecting a single lobe with strong suspicion of MAKP.

- A circumscribed cystic lesion in the air, a simple suspicion of MAKP and persistent fever having been operated on by lobectomy (which explains the number of false positives (13/14) in our series).

CHAPTER II
OBSERVATIONS

OBSERVATION 1

The infant (B.R.) was female, 50 days old, with a history of prematurity of 32 weeks' amenorrhoea and a neonatal weight of 1550 g, having been hospitalised at birth for 29 days for maternal-foetal infection and then at 40 days for respiratory distress. On physical examination, polypnoea at 45 cycles per minute, chest indrawing, xiphoid funnelling and an oxygen saturation of 82% on room air were found. The chest X-ray showed hyper-aeration of the right pulmonary hemi-field with right pulmonary distension, trans-mediastinal herniation and mediastinal deviation to the left **(Fig. 1)**.

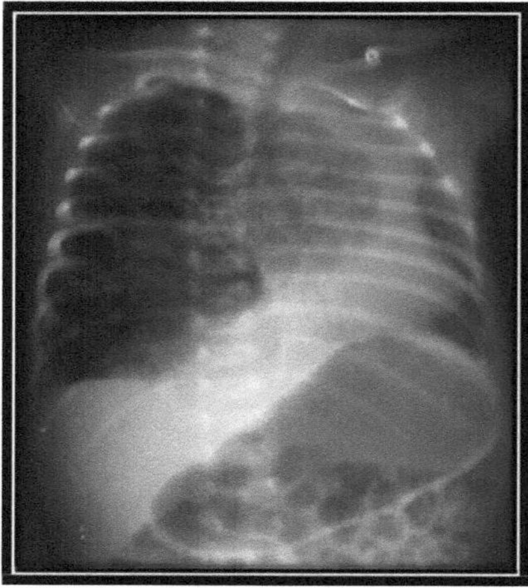

Figure 1: Front chest X-ray: hyper-aeration of the right lung, trans-mediastinal hernia, deviation of the mediastinal elements to the left.

Chest CT showed significant distension of the right upper and middle lobes due to the coalescence of multiple air bubbles. The right lower lobe was collapsed, pressed against the spine, and the mediastinum was pushed to the left, with reduced ventilation of the left lung **(Fig. 2)**. The multi-cystic appearance of the lesion led to the diagnosis of MAKP of the right upper and middle lobes.

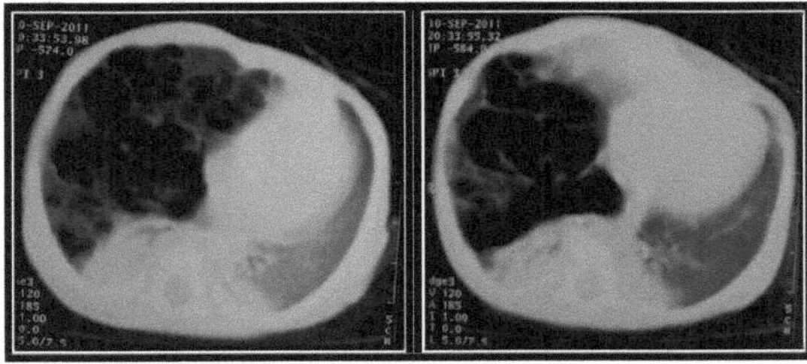

Figure 2: Chest CT scan: multiple air cysts in the right upper and middle lobes.

A perfusion lung scan performed when there was doubt about congenital lobar emphysema showed hypoperfusion in the right upper lobe **(Fig. 3)**.The infant was operated on at t h e age of 55 days by right posterolateral thoracotomy. The intra-operative appearance was that of MAKP involving the right upper and middle lobes. The lesser scissure was not iden-ified. An upper and middle bilobectomy was performed. Immediately post-operatively, with a haemoglobin level of 6.1 g.$^{dl-1}$, a transfusion of 40 mL of phenotyped blood was performed. The chest tube was removed 2 days after the operation. The infant w a s handed over to his parents on D5 post-operatively.On section, the surgical specimen showed multiple cystic lumens, the largest of which measured 1 cm in diameter.

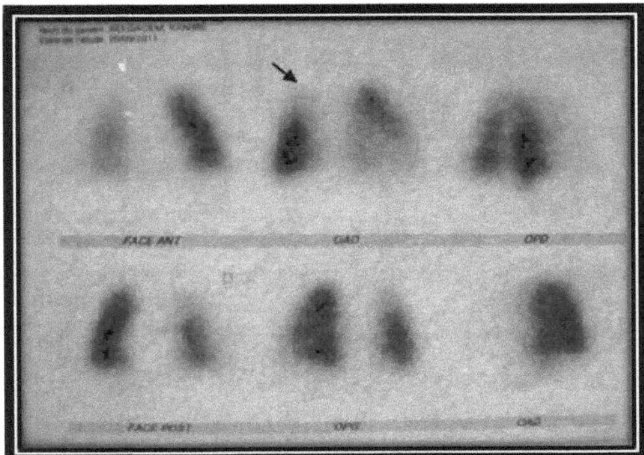

Figure 3: Lung perfusion scintigraphy: hypo-perfusion of the right upper lobe

Histologically, these were multiple optically empty cystic cavities of variable size with no epithelial lining of their own, surrounded in places by a giant cell reaction. These cysts were located in the septa separating the lobules. The alveoli, bronchi and bronchioles w e r e normal in appearance. This was consistent with **pulmonary interstitial emphysema (Fig. 4)**.

The follow-up was 30 months. The infant presented with recurrent bronchopneumonia and retained an asymmetric left hemithorax.

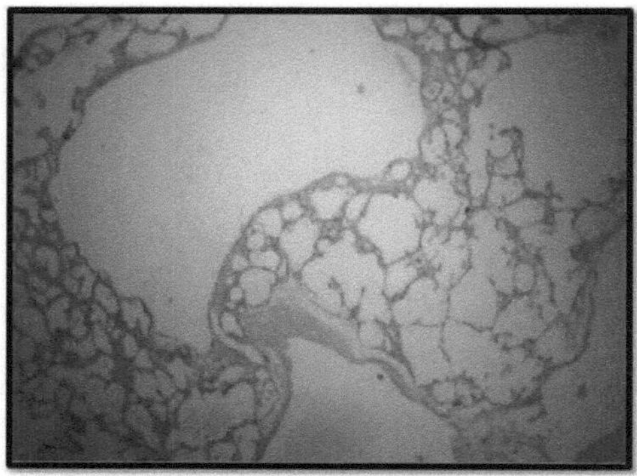

Figure 4: Histology of pulmonary interstitial emphysema

OBSERVATION 2

The newborn baby (B.Y.) was female, 23 days old, the result of a normal pregnancy, carried to term with a neonatal weight of 2750 g and who presented respiratory distress at the age of 3 days.Examination revealed a polypnoeic newborn with a Silvermann score of 2, with heart sounds more audible on the right. The chest X-ray showed a total left pneumothorax, with passive atelectasis of the homolateral lung parenchyma and rightward displacement of the mediastinum **(Fig. 5)**.

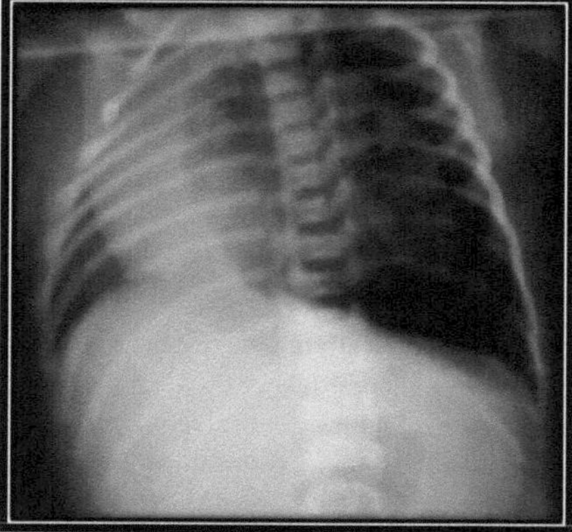

Figure 5: Front chest X-ray: left total and compressive pneumothorax with deviation of the mediastinum to the right.

The chest CT scan also showed cystic aeri of variable size in the left lower lobe, which was retracted. The right lung was compressed **(Fig. 6)**.

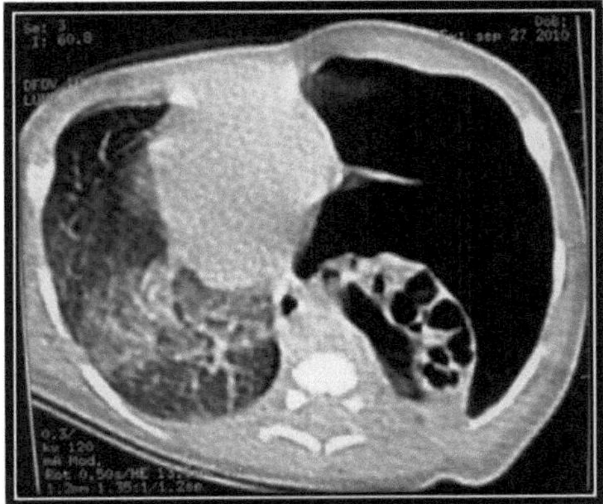

Figure 6. Chest CT scan: cystic aerial images of the left lower lobe.

After exsufflation of the pneumothorax, it recurred, necessitating placement of a left pleural drain, which remained in place for 7 days. Radiological examination showed the persistence of clear cystic images of the left lower lobe **(Fig. 7)**.A new chest CT scan was ordered, which showed an appearance suggestive of MAKP of the left lower lobe **(Fig. 8)**. Doppler ultrasound showed no systemic vessels vascularising the malformation.

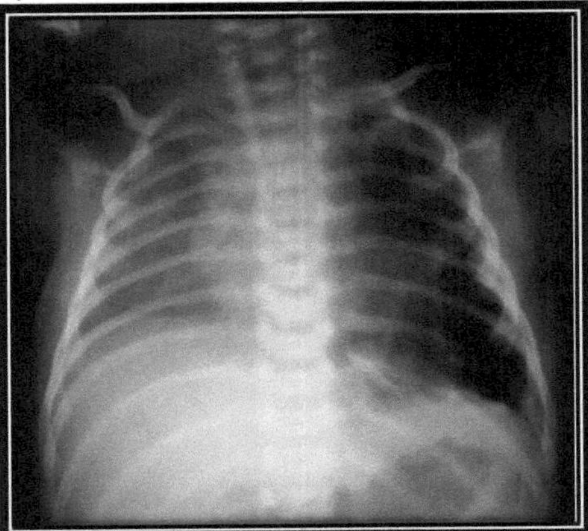

Figure 7. Front chest X-ray after removal of chest drainage: clear images of the left lower lobe.

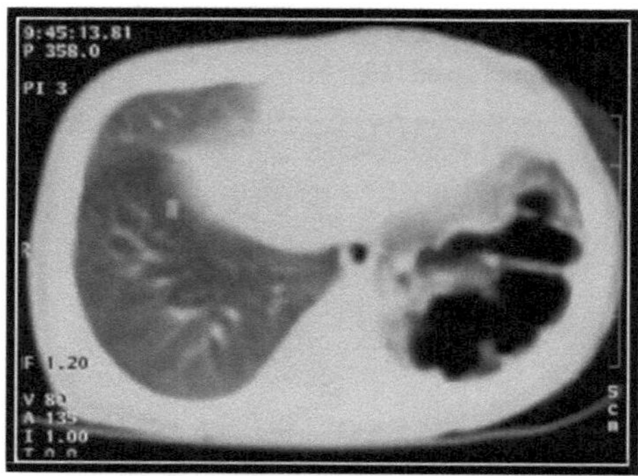

Figure 8. Chest CT scan: appearance of MAKP in the left lower lobe.

The newborn was operated on at the age of 23 days via a left thoracotomy at the 5th intercostal space. Exploration revealed multiple pleural adhesions, particularly in the lower lobe. The lower lobe was the site of numerous cystic formations ranging in size from 0.2 to 2 cm **(Fig. 9)**.

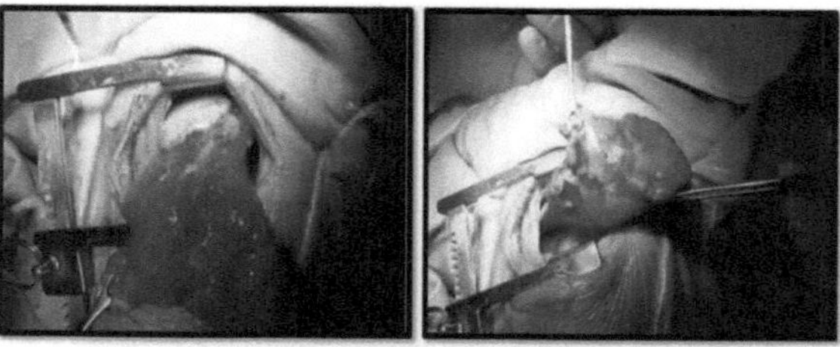

Figure 9. Intraoperative appearance.

A left lower lobectomy was performed **(Fig. 10)**.

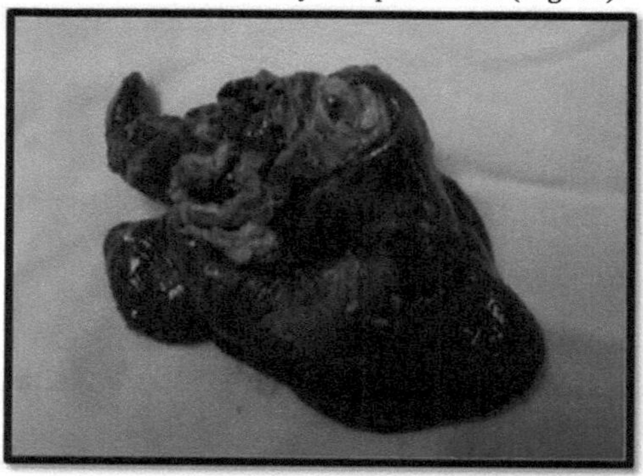

Figure 10. Left lower lobectomy specimen

The course was marked by the onset of fever on D-1 post-op and a CRP of 123 mg.$^{L-1}$, necessitating treatment with Cefotaxime and Amikacin. The chest tube was removed on D-4 post-op, and the hospital stay was 27 days.On sectioning of the operative specimen, there was a cystic formation measuring 5 cm in diameter with a whitish pasty content.Histologically, the cystic formation contained eosinophilic material with ghostly vascular structures. This necrotic material was unusual in that it was rich in keratin lamellae, as is usually seen in the alveoli of the foetus at the end of pregnancy.This cystic cavity, which was sub pleural in topography, corresponded to a focus of pulmonary infarction that was undergoing detersion, as evidenced by the presence of a large macrophagic and giant cell reaction around the cavity.The presence of keratin lamellae in this focus indicates that this infarction occurred antenatally.The lung tissue surrounding this lesion included sections of arteries with thrombosed lumens and organised repermeabilised or calcified thrombi.The histological diagnosis was that of **a** detaching ante-natal **pulmonary infarction (Fig. 11)**. The subsequent course was favourable with a 3.5-year follow-up. The follow-up chest X-ray showed good expansion of the left lung **(Fig. 12)**.

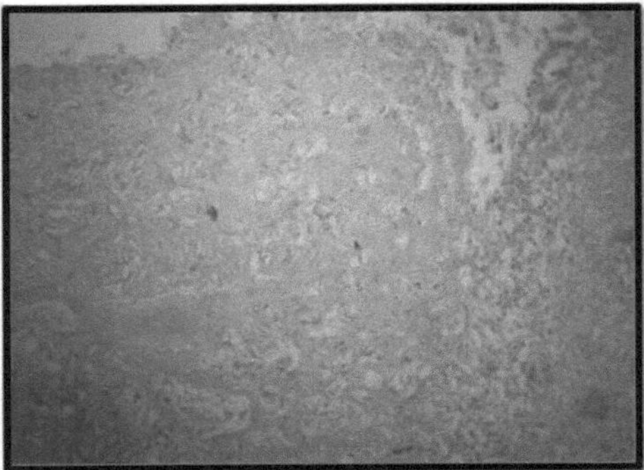

Figure 11. Histology: antenatal pulmonary infarction (keratin lamellae indicate antenatal origin).

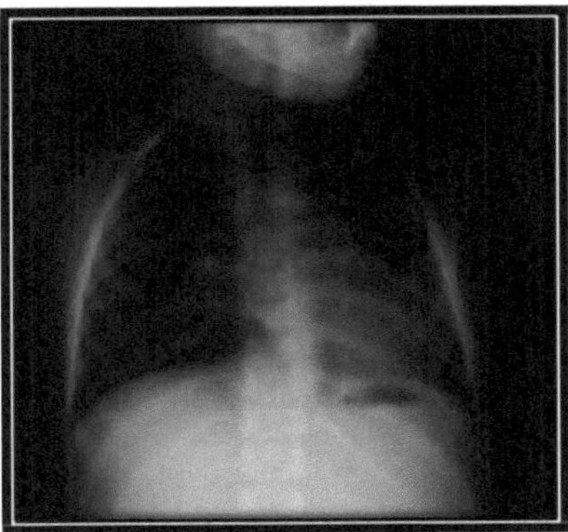

Figure 12. Radiograph chest of X-ray: good lung expansion.

OBSERVATION 3

A 15-month-old male infant (C.M.) was admitted to hospital at the age of 10 months with a cough and fever. He was diagnosed with a right lung abscess and treated with clavulanic acid. During his outpatient follow-up, a chest X-ray taken outside the infectious episode showed a rounded, hyper-clear formation 8 cm long, occupying the right pulmonary hemi-chamber.

A thoracic CT scan revealed a sequellar cavity in the right lower lobe. The diagnosis was MAKP of the right upper lobe and the infant was operated on by right thoracotomy at the 4th intercostal space. Intraoperative exploration revealed a very thickened and adherent pleura in all 3 lobes, and particularly in the upper lobe, which showed a cystic formation. Puncture of this cyst returned air, allowing temporary deflation of the lobe. A right upper lobectomy was performed. The hospital stay was 5 days.

Macroscopic examination of the surgical specimen revealed a unilocular cyst measuring 6 cm in diameter. Histologically, the cyst had a thick, fibrous wall with no epithelial lining. In places, this wall was lined with macrophagic cells, including foreign-body type giant cells. Outside the cyst, the parenchyma was in places the site of an interstitial and intra-alveolar inflammatory infiltrate.

The visceral pleura was thickened and fibrous, suggesting **a cyst following a neonatal pulmonary infarction.**

After 6 months, the child was asymptomatic.
N.B. The images and X-rays have not been found in the archives.

OBSERVATION 4

An 18-month-old female infant (S.I.) from a full-term pregnancy complicated by intrauterine growth retardation, who had presented with recurrent bronchopneumonia without fever since the age of 6 months.

The chest X-ray showed a well-limited, homogeneous, right lower lobar clearness measuring approximately 7 cm in long axis **(Fig. 13)**.

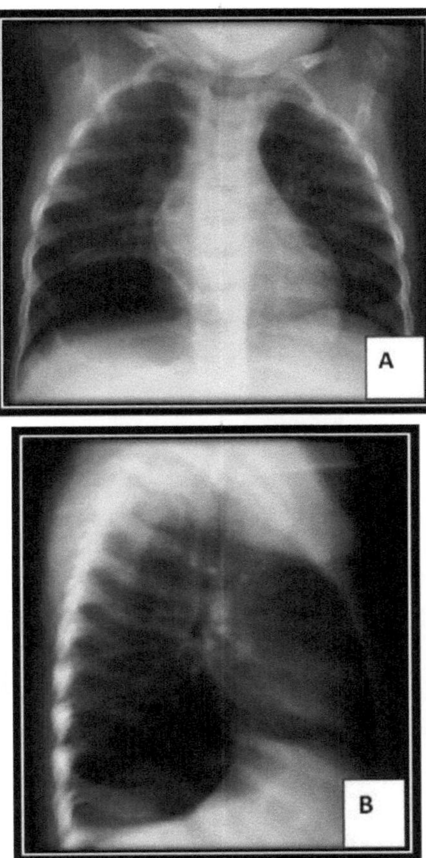

Figure 13. A: Front chest X-ray: well circumscribed right lower lobe. **B:** Profile chest X-ray: right lower lobe with posterior projection.

TOGD revealed supracarinal gastro-oesophageal reflux without hiatal hernia **(Fig. 14)**. Chest CT showed a large, homogeneous, well-limited, thin-walled, aerotic, right lower lobar cystic formation measuring 7x6 cm. The appearance was consistent with right lower lobe PKA **(Fig. 15)**.

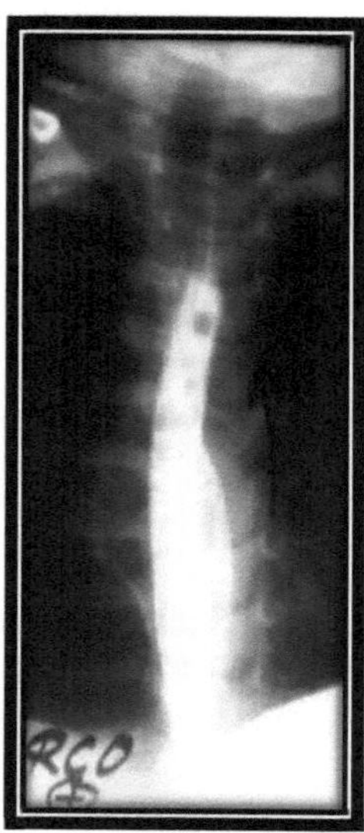

Figure 14. Massive gastro-oesophageal reflux.

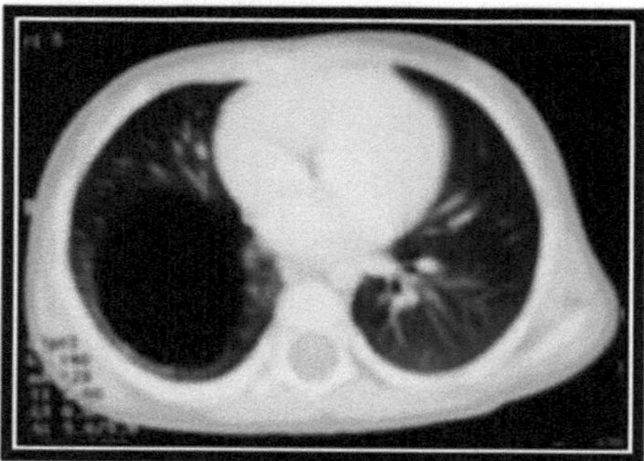

Figure 15. Chest CT scan: unilocular cystic formation in the right lower lobe.

The infant was operated on via a right thoracotomy at the 6th intercostal space. Intra-operative examination revealed a right lower lobe which was very enlarged, with a large multi-cystic formation at its base measuring 7 cm in length. The rest of the lung parenchyma, mainly the nelson, was probably dysplastic. A right lower lobectomy was performed with the formation removed **(Fig. 16)**.

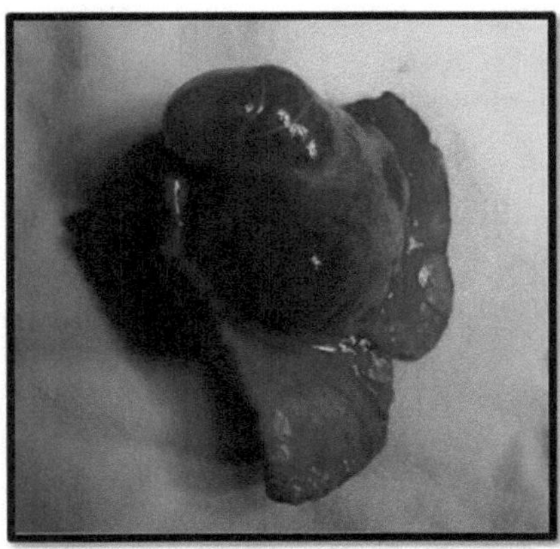

Figure 16. Right lower lobectomy specimen.

The post-operative course was straightforward and the infant was handed over to his parents on D4 post-op.Macroscopic examination of the operative specimen confirmed the existence of a subpleural cystic formation with a thickened wall and aerated content measuring 6 cm in diameter. The rest of the lung tissue was congestive and collapsed in places. Histclogically, the cyst had a wall made of fibrous tissue with few cells, and with no epithelial liıing. The cyst wall was separated from the lung parenchyma by a band of loose connective tissue with haemorrhagic suffusions. The cyst raised a thickened, fibrous visceral pleura. The rest of the lung tissue showed foci of atelectasis and focal areas of cubic metaplasia of the alveolar lining, as well as a nodular lymphocytic infiltrate **(Fig. 17)**.

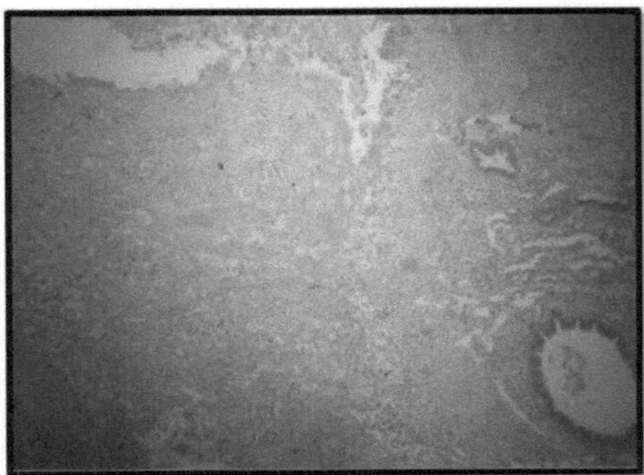

Figure 17. Histology: post-natal pulmonary infarction.

This appearance is that of **a cyst secondary to a post-natal pulmonary infarction** of the right lower lobe.One year later, the course was marked by recurrent bronchopneumonia and asthmatic dyspnoea, most likely related to gastro-oesophageal reflux.

OBSERVATION 5

The girl (J.G.), aged 4, with no notable pathological history, presented with haemoptoic sputum without fever or change in general condition, which had been present for 2 years and had been progressively worsening for 2 months. The physical examination was unremarkable.

Hydatid serology, tuberculin intradermal reaction (IDR) and Koch's bacillus tests on 3 consecutive days were negative. The chest X-ray showed an alveolar opacity, poorly limited to the right paracardium **(Fig. 18)**.

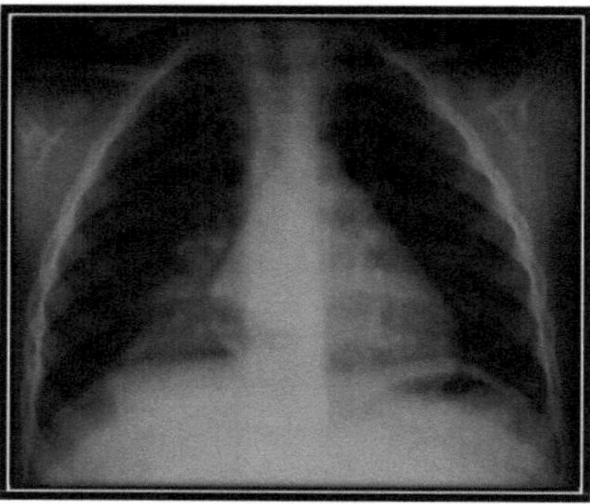

Figure 18. Chest X-ray: right paracardiac opacity.

A complementary thoracic CT scan concluded that there was a focus of parenchymal condensation, postero-basal on the right, 5 cm long, containing multiple centimetre-sized cystic lesions of heterogeneous density suggestive of MAKP or pulmonary sequestration **(Fig. 19)**.

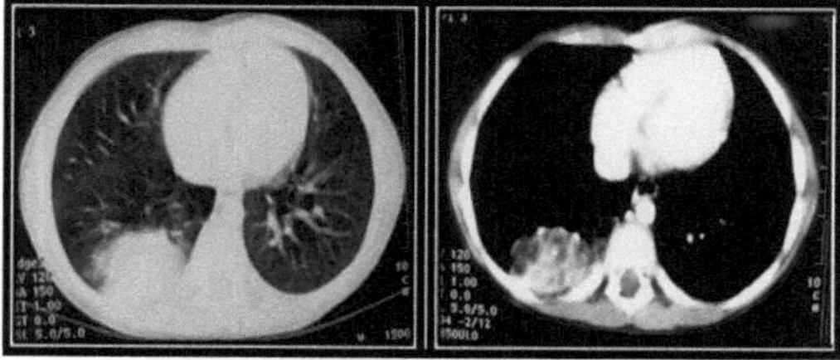

Figure 19. Chest CT: right posterobasal parenchymal condensation: MAKP or pulmonary sequestration?

Thoracic Doppler ultrasound did not reveal any systemic feeder vessels. The child underwent thoracotomy to the 5th right intercostal space. Exploration revealed an unventilated, indurated basal pyramid, the manipulation of which caused pus to leak through the endotracheal intubation tube. There were also multiple mediastinal adenopathies. The intraoperative appearance was that of a right lower lobe MAKP **(Fig. 20)**. A right lower lobectomy was performed **(Fig. 21)** and antibiotic prophylaxis with clavulanic acid was initiated. The post-operative course was straightforward. The 2 thoracic drains were removed on D-3 and D-5 post-operatively. The child was handed over to his parents on D-7 post-operatively. Macroscopically, the surgical specimen showed a purplish posterior basal area. On cross-section, the bronchi and bronchioles at this level had a thickened wall and dilated lumen. This bronchial dilatation was associated with a parenchymal condensation. The lumen of one bronchus contained a brownish, hard, thread-like foreign body.

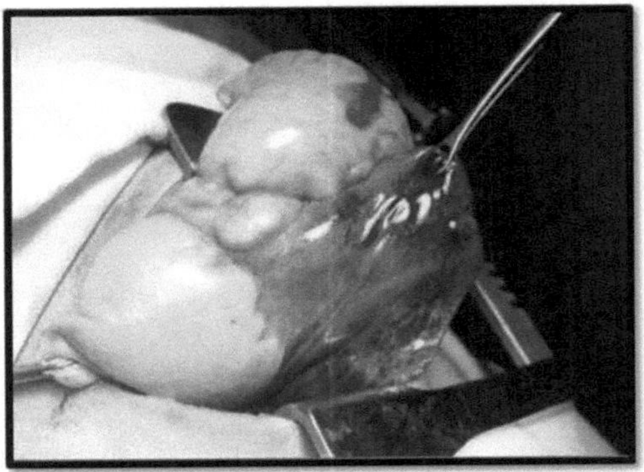

Figure 20. Intraoperative appearance of MAKP in the right lower lobe.

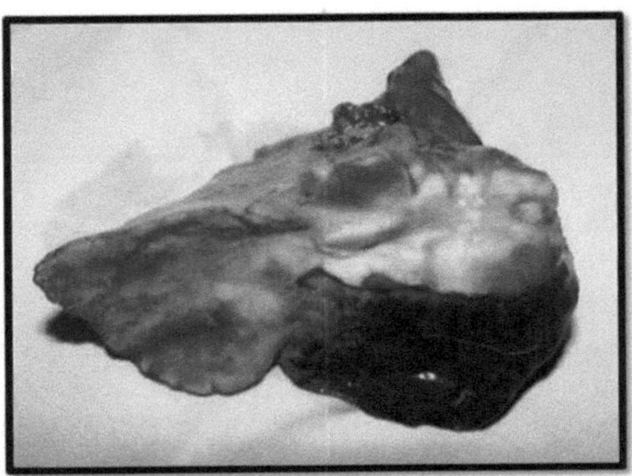

Figure 21. Right lower lobectomy specimen.

Histologically, the posterobasal segment showed dilatation of the bronchi and bronchioles, which often had a pus-filled lumen and ulcerated mucosa. The lung tissue around these bronchi w a s often the site of an abundant, polymorphous inflammatory infiltrate. Microscopic examination confirmed the presence of a foreign body of plant origin in the lumen of a bronchus.Anatomopathological examination of the surgical specimen concluded that **there were lesions of bronchial dilatation** in suppurated places, secondary to a plant foreign body, involving the postero-basal segment of the right lower lobe. The subsequent outcome was favourable, with resolution of the haemoptysis.

OBSERVATION 6

A female infant (T.M.), aged 3 months and 8 days, who had presented with recurrent bronchopneumonia and dyspnoea in a febrile setting since the age of 1 month. Under antibiotic therapy, the course was marked by a recurrence of respiratory symptoms with worsening dyspnoea progressing to respiratory distress requiring respiratory assistance for 10 days. The chest X-ray showed a watery opacity occupying almost the entire left lung field, with the mediastinum pushing back to the right **(Fig. 22)**.

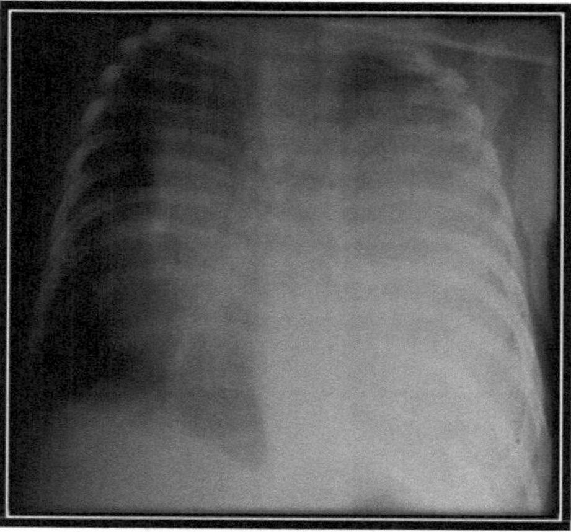

Figure 22. Front chest X-ray: opacity involving the left lung, with deviation of the mediastinum to the right.

Thoracic angioscan showed a left lower lobe distended by several cystic formations with mediastinal displacement, with no systemic artery. The appearance was suggestive of MAKP of the left lower lobe **(Fig. 23)**.

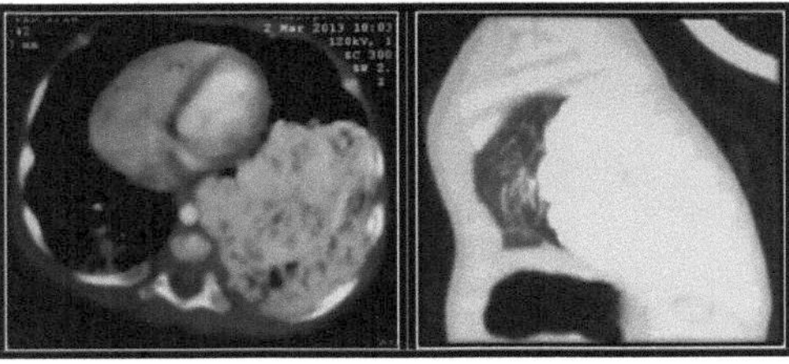

Figure 23. Thoracic angioscan: cystic formation in the left lower lobe: MAKP?

Cardiac Doppler ultrasound was normal.

A left thoracotomy to the 5th intercostal space was performed. Intraoperative exploration revealed a thickened visceral pleura. The left lower lobe was the site of an enormous reddish-brown, non-ventilated formation, which appeared to be hyper-vascularised, 12 cm long with no systemic vessels **(Fig. 24)**.

A left lower lobectomy was performed.

Macroscopic examination of the operative specimen revealed a large section of the left lower lobe with a hepatic appearance, a few haemorrhagic foci and a peripheral cavity measuring 1 cm **(Fig. 25)**. Histologically, the hepatic appearance was consistent with a benign, multifocal vascular tumour involving the inter-alveolar septa and the rest of the interstitial tissue. This proliferation consisted of capillaries with mostly reduced lumen. These capillaries were lined with regular endothelial cells showing some evidence of mitosis. The tumour was sometimes visible in the The walls of the veins were dilated. The haemorrhagic areas were related to ischaemic necrosis lesions. The cyst noted macroscopically corresponded to a bronchiole with significant cystic dilatation and a widely ulcerated wall.

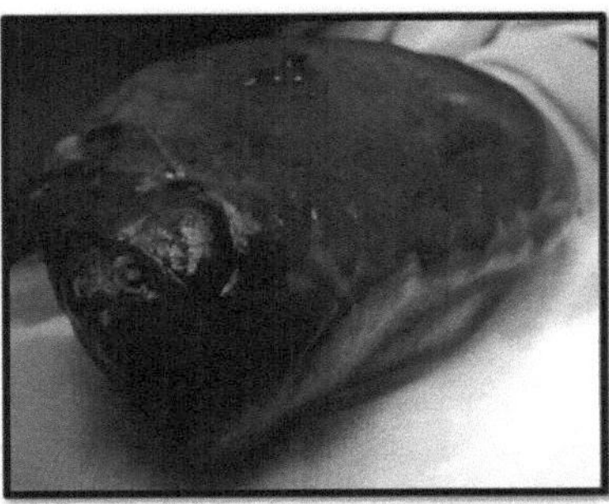

Figure 24. Intraoperative appearance: hyper-vascularised formation of the left lower lobe.

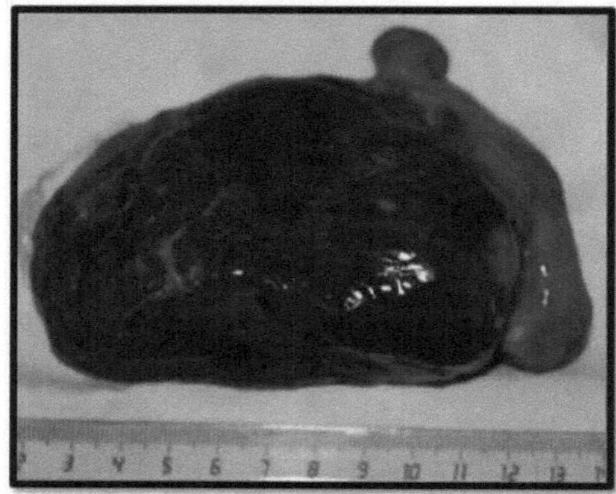

Figure 25. Macroscopic appearance of the surgical specimen: left lower lobe with hepatic appearance.

Pathological examination concluded that the patient had pulmonary capillary haemangiomatosis of the left lower lobe **(Fig. 26)**. The patient died at 7 days post-operatively as a result of a nosocomial infection.

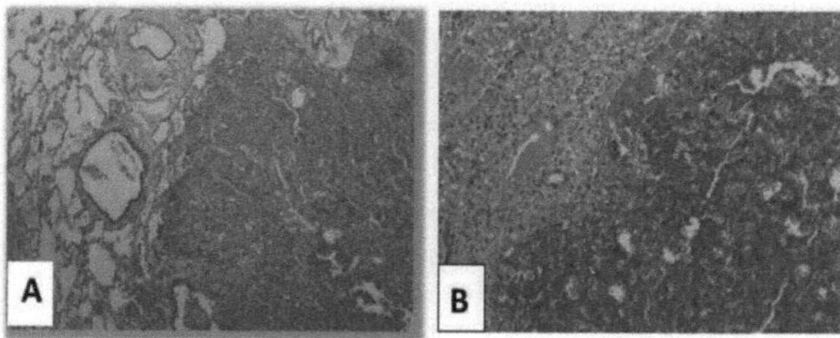

Figure 26. Histology. **A:** Diffuse capillary proliferation involving the inter-alveolar septa. **B:** Ischaemic and haemorrhagic necrosis.

OBSERVATION 7

The female infant (B.A.), aged 2 months and 9 days, the result of a normal pregnancy carried to term, presented 15 days prior to hospitalisation with a cough, dyspnoea and fever unimproved by Clavulanic Acid-based antibiotic therapy. Physical examination revealed a fever of 38.5°C, polypnoea at 45 cycles per minute with signs of struggle, decreased vesicular murmurs on the right and bilateral snoring rales on pulmonary auscultation. The chest X-ray showed a hydroaerobic opacity of approximately 10 cm long axis involving the lower two-thirds of the right lung field without mediastinal displacement **(Fig. 27)**.

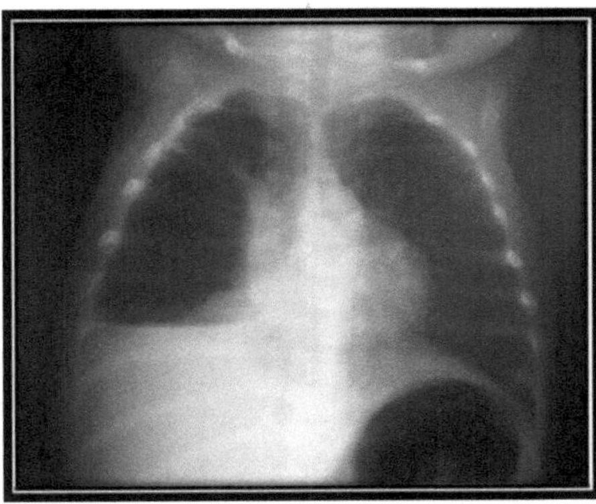

Figure 27-1 Front upright chest X-ray: hyperclarity of the lower two-thirds of the right lung field with hydroaerobic level

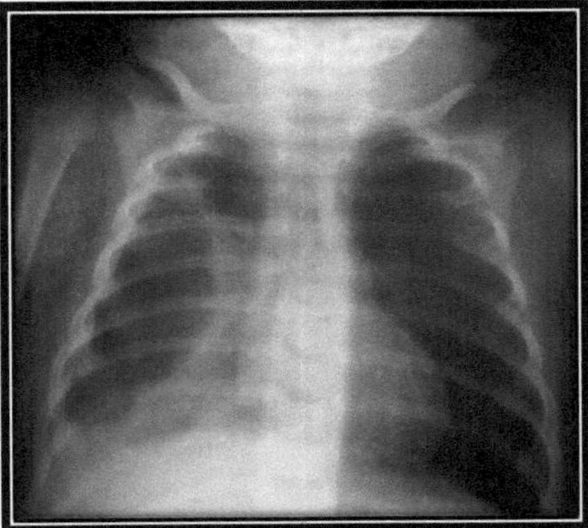

Figure 27-2. Prone radiograph of the chest: hyperclarity of most of the outer part of the right pulmonary hemi-field with filling of the pleural cul-de-sac.

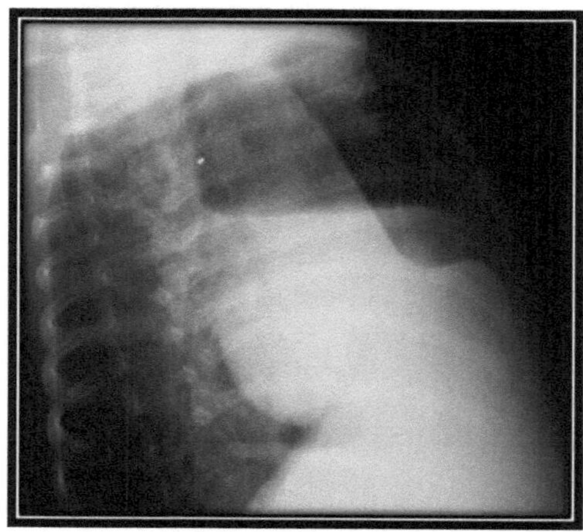

Figure 27-3. Radiograph of the chest in profile: hydro-aeroid opacity with anterior projection.

A thoracic CT scan confirmed the existence of a clean-walled collection measuring 9x7x5 cm occupying the right medio-thoracic part, with hydro-aeric content, appearing to continue with pleural effusion from the large cavity and signs of parenchymal compression of the lower and middle lobes **(Fig. 28)**.

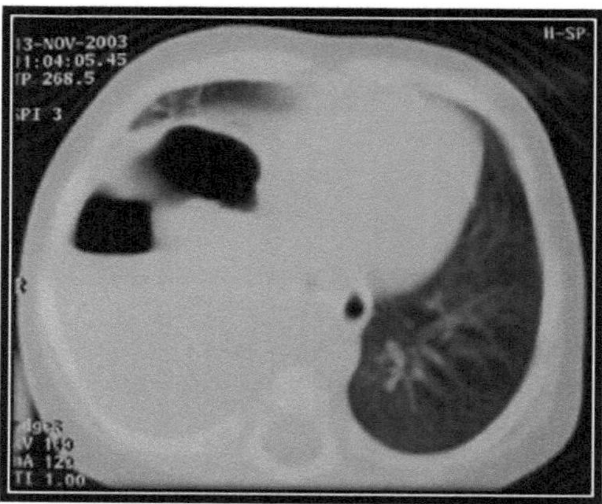

Figure 28. Chest CT scan: hydroaerobic collection occupying the right lung hemifield.

The infant was operated on via a right posterobasal thoracotomy to the 4th intercostal space. Exploration revealed a highly inflammatory parietal and visceral pleura **(Fig. 29)**. Aspiration yielded 150 ml of thick yellowish pus, which was removed for bacteriological examination **(Fig. 30)**.

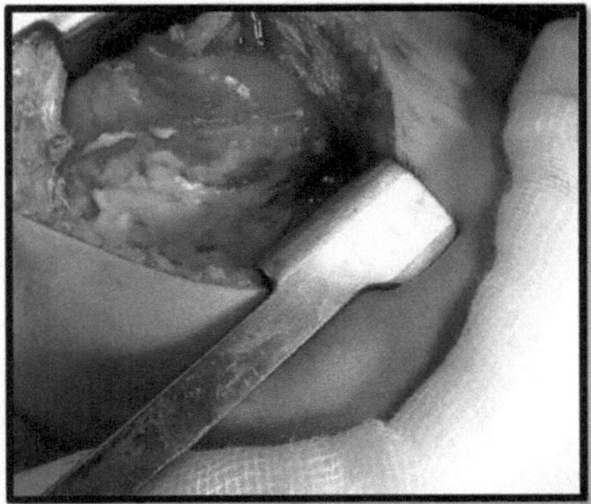

Figure 29. Intraoperative investigation: highly inflamed parietal and visceral pleura

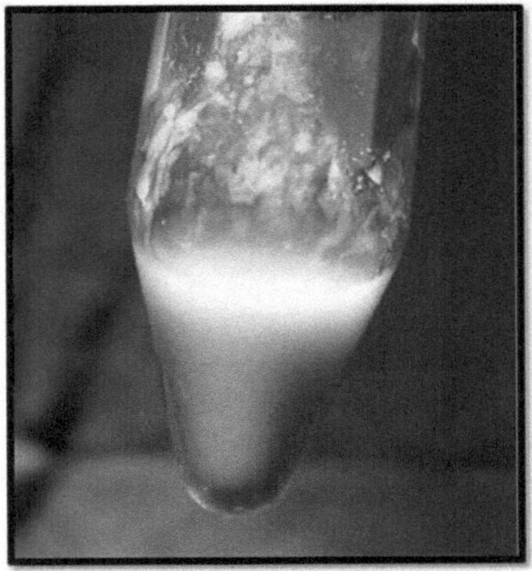

Figure 30. Pus sampling.

On examination of the right lower lobe, there were 2 cystic bubbling formations located in the apical segment and the basal pyramid. A right lower lobectomy was performed **(Fig. 31)**.

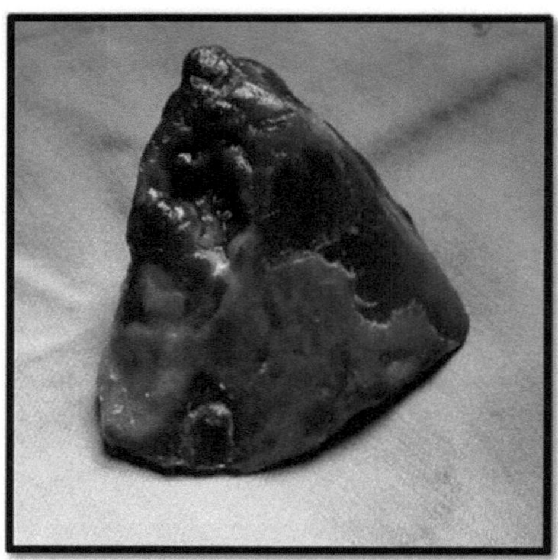

Figure 31. Right lower lobectomy specimen.

Bacteriological examination of the pleural fluid revealed Staphylococcus Aureus Meti-S, and the infant was treated with appropriate antibiotics. Post-operative management was straightforward.Macroscopic examination of the operative specimen revealed a lung lobe measuring 5x4x3 cm, covered mainly at the base with thick false membranes. On section, there was a cystic cavity measuring 1 cm in long axis, open at the surface. Another cystic cavity measuring 8 mm was found close to the lobar bronchus. Histologically, the 2 cavities had purulent contents and were surrounded by a border of granulation tissue reminiscent of the pyogenic membrane seen around abscesses. Elsewhere, the lung tissue was normal in appearance. In particular, there was no inflammation. The pleura was lined with large fibrino-leukocytic deposits. Pathological examination concluded that there were **2 pulmonary abscesses**, 1 of which was peripheral and fistulised with a large fibrinous pleuritis. The follow-up was 1 month. The patient was subsequently lost to follow-up.

OBSERVATION 8

A 14-month-old male infant (A.A.), with no notable personal history, presented 2 months ago with a dry cough and fever that had refused symptomatic and antibiotic treatment. Physical examination revealed a reduction in left vesicular murmurs. The chest X-ray showed a homogeneous, oval, 8x5 c m , upper left lobar opacity of watery tone, surmounted by a hydro-aeric level **(Fig. 32)**. A complementary thoracic CT confirmed the existence of a cystic mass containing a hydro-aeroid level, with a thick, regular wall, involving most of the left upper lobe **(Fig. 33)**.An inflammatory syndrome persisted, with white blood cells at 19,000 mm3.mL-1 and a CRP of 150 mg.L-1 after 13 days of antibiotic therapy. The infant was operated on via a thoracotomy to the 4th left intercostal space. Intraoperative examination revealed a thickened pleura, numerous haemorrhagic adhesions over the left upper lobe and large mediastinal adenopathies measuring 1 to 2.5 cm in diameter.

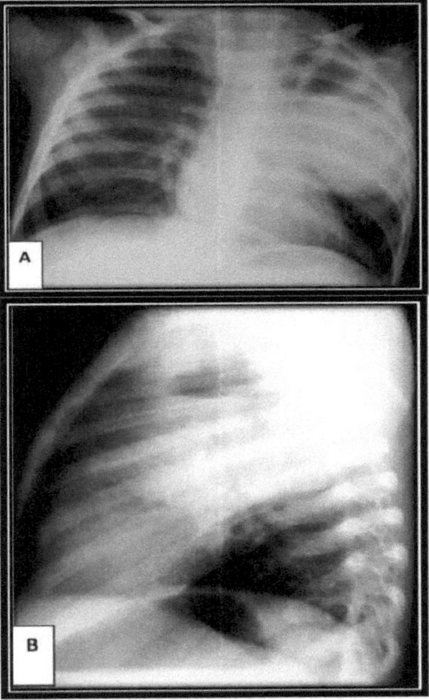

Figure 32. A: Front chest X-ray: opacity of the left upper lobe surmounted by a hydro-aeric level. **B:** Chest X-ray, profile: left upper lobar opacity with a hydro-aeric level, posterior projection.

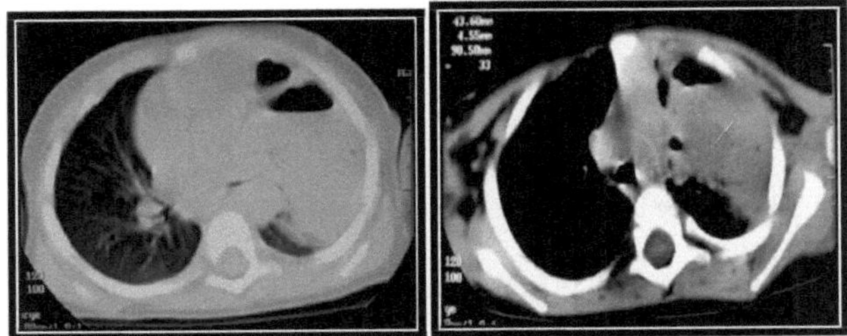

Figure 33. Chest CT: cystic mass in the left upper lobe with hydroaerobic level.

Most of the left upper lobe was taken up by a purulent cystic formation. A left upper lobectomy was performed **(Fig. 34)**.

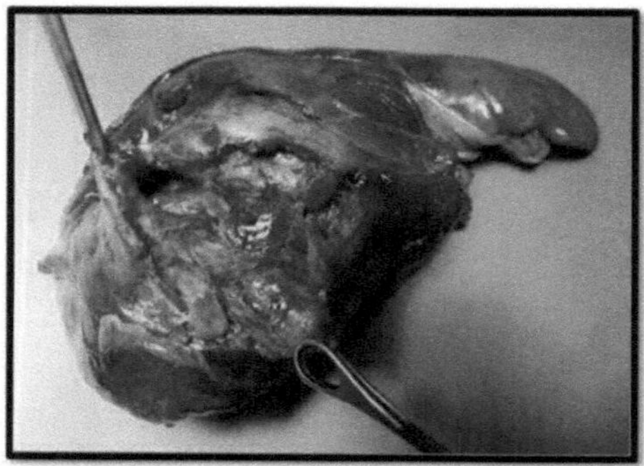

Figure 34. Left upper lobectomy specimen.

Antibiotic prophylaxis was based on Cefotaxime.

The post-operative course was straightforward, with removal of the chest tube at 4 days post-operatively. The infant was handed over to his parents the following day. Macroscopically, the lobectomy specimen measured 10x5x3 cm with a brownish surface and an empty cystic cavity 1.2 cm long. On section, the parenchyma had a brownish appearance and contained a 2nd cystic cavity 3 cm long, communicating with the one initially described. Histologically, the cavities had a relatively thick wall made up of 2 layers: an inner one resembling a fleshy bud and an outer one made up of connective tissue relatively rich in fibroblast-type cells. This wall appearance is very similar to that of the pyogenic membrane surrounding abscesses. However, the lung tissue did not show any histological lesions, leading to the conclusion that **it was an abscess of the left upper lobe.** The follow-up was 1 month. The patient was lost to follow-up.

OBSERVATION 9

A female infant (A.H.), aged three and a half months, who presented one week prior to hospitalisation with febrile bronchopneumonia, treated with clavulanic acid. A chest X-ray showed a well-limited opacity in the right upper lobe **(Fig. 35).**

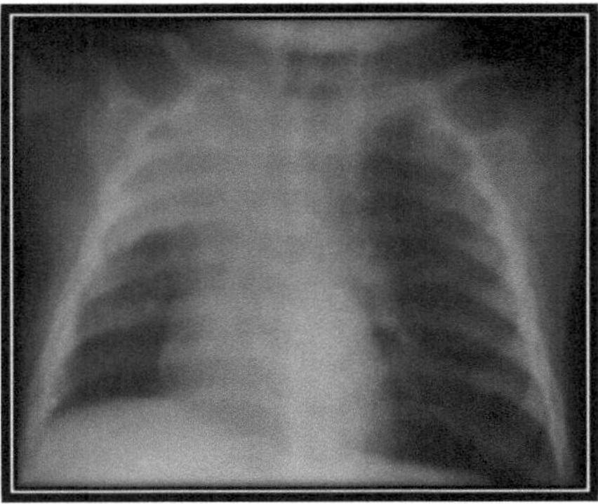

Figure 35. Front chest X-ray: opacity of the right upper lobe.

Progression under medical treatment was marked by a progressive worsening. Radiological examination after the infant had been put on antibiotics showed that the opacity had become heterogeneous and aerated, with the appearance of a pleural effusion **(Fig. 36)**.

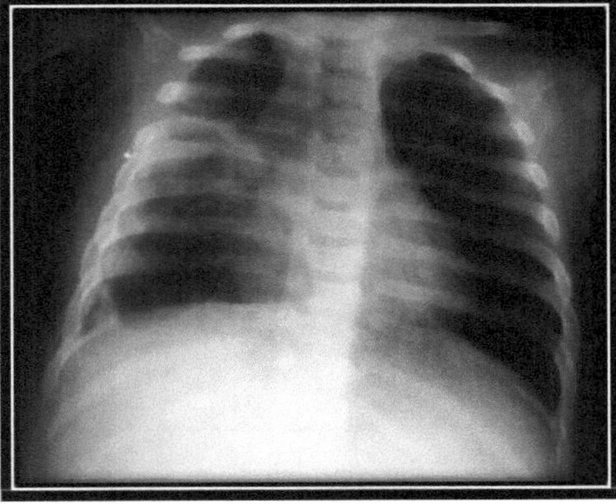

Figure 36. Check control: opacity heterogeneous aerated with filling of the right pleural pouch.

Given the dyspnoea, fever and biological signs of infection (CRP 252 mg.L^{-1}; hyper-leukocytosis 49,000 $mm3.mL-1$), the initial antibiotic treatment was changed to a combination of Cefotaxime and Vancomycin. A thoracic CT scan was ordered, and showed a 5 cm, thin-walled, regular, cystic, hydroaerobic, parenchymal formation in the right upper lobe. This was associated with a 2nd small cystic formation in the same lobe, with the presence o f a cloistered pleural effusion and atelectasis of the right middle and lower lobes. The diagnosis of right upper lobar MAKP associated with a septated pleural effusion was accepted and the infant was operated on by a right posterolateral thoracotomy. The parietal pleura was very thickened and completely adherent to the visceral pleura. Investigation revealed haemorrhagic fluid between the 2 pleura and a purulent collection in the lower pouch. Dissection revealed and evacuated a 1st purulent collection in the right upper lobar region, 5 cm long, and a 2nd, smaller cystic cavity in the upper lobar region, 2 cm in diameter **(Fig. 37)**. A right upper lobectomy was performed **(Fig. 38)**.

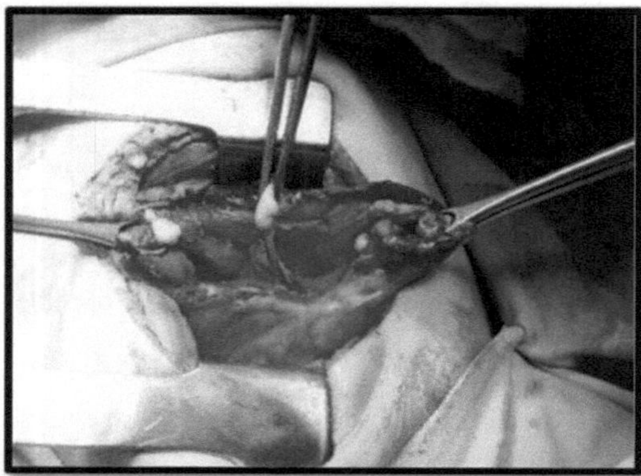

Figure 37. Intraoperative appearance: 2 cystic cavities in the right upper lobe.

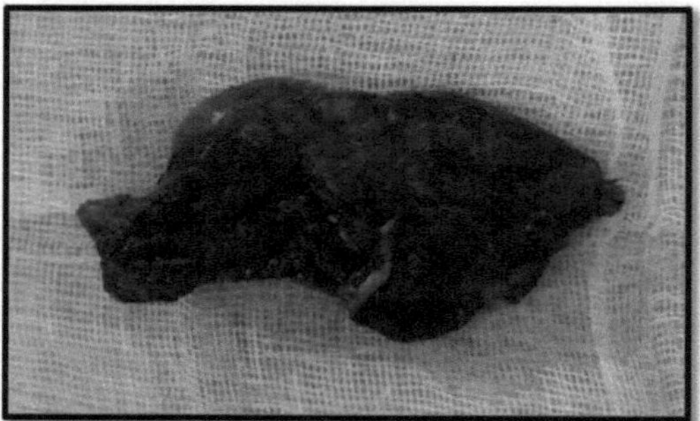

Figure 38. Right upper lobectomy specimen.

Per-operative antibiotic prophylaxis was carried out with Cefazolin. Bacteriological examination of the pleural fluid was negative. The post-operative course was straightforward, with the chest tube removed at 5 days post-operatively, and the infant handed over to his parents at 13 days post-operatively.Macroscopic examination of the operative specimen revealed a brownish fragment of lung tissue measuring 7x4x2 cm with 2 contiguous cystic cavities on cross-section, the largest of which was 2 cm long. Elsewhere, the lung tissue contained multiple yellowish-white foci measuring between 0.2 and 0.5 cm. Histologically, the 2 cystic cavities were bordered by granulation tissue covered on the surface by fibrino-leukocytic material and formed by capillary-type blood vessels and an abundant polymorphic inflammatory infiltrate with no epithelial structure. Elsewhere, the lung parenchyma showed foci in which the alveoli contained numerous macrophages, sometimes associated with neutrophil polynuclei. The small bronchi and bronchioles were of normal morphology. Histological examination revealed no pathogenic agent and concluded that **the patient had abscessed right upper lobe lung disease.** The subsequent course was marked by a single episode of cough without fever, treated symptomatically, and the follow-up was 1? months.

COMMENT 10

The 40-day-old male infant (S.F.), born during a normal pregnancy with a morphological ultrasound scan that came back without any abnormality, presented at t h e age cf 28 days with a fever of 39°C with no respiratory signs or other complaints. The urine cytobacteriological examination was positive, and the fever was initially attributed to the urinary tract infection and treated with antibiotics. The blood count showed a hyper-leukocytosis of 23600 per mL. The chest X-ray showed an excavated opacity covering most of the right hemithorax, with only the apex and the costodiaphragmatic cul de sac present **(Fig. 39).**

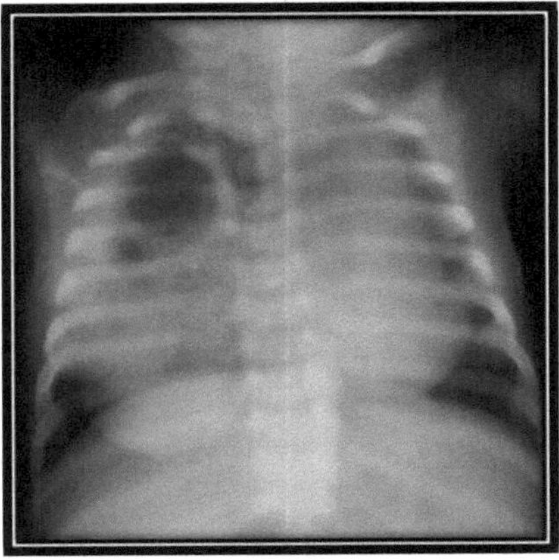

Figure 39. Front chest X-ray: excavated opacity of the hemi right thorax.

At the age of 33 days, the newborn presented with a cough without fever and a normal somatic examination. Thoracic ultrasound showed a large bilobed cystic formation with a thick, clean wall, finely echogenic content, containing reverberating air echoes. Chest CT showed a large, thick-walled, bilobed cystic mass, mainly posterior, measuring 6x5x4 cm. This formation was contrast-enhanced at the periphery and contained a few air bubbles, an appearance compatible with a malformative origin **(Fig. 40).**

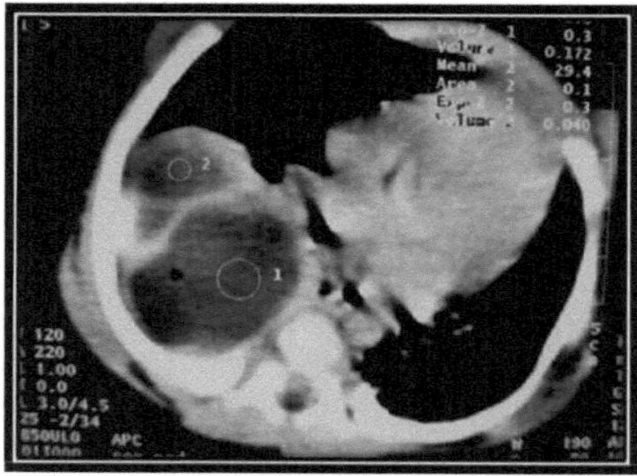

Figure 40. Chest CT scan: bilobed cystic mass in the right lung.

TOGD showed no oesophageal communication with the mass. The newborn was operated on at the age of 40 days by a posterolateral right thoracotomy. Intraoperative exploration revealed a thickened parietal pleura and a right lung that was unrecognisable because it was not ventilating. There were 3 pulmonary cystic formations **(Fig. 41)**.

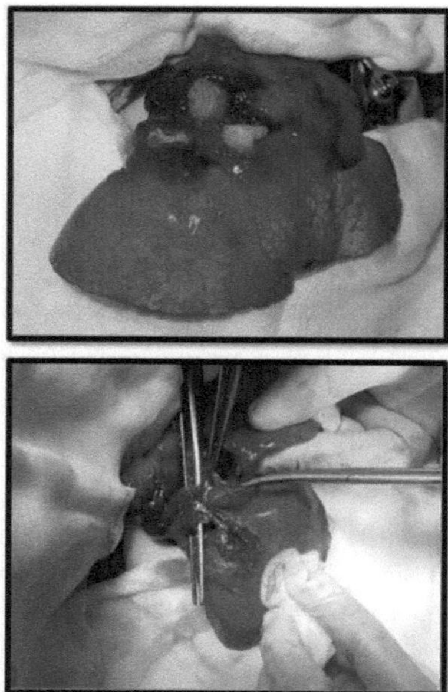

Figure 41. Intraoperative appearance: 3 cystic formations involving the 3 right lobes.

Puncture of these formations yielded pus **(Fig. 42)**. Each of these formations was about 5 cm long and was located very close to the junction between the greater and lesser scissures. After evacuation, the formations in the upper and lower lobes were found to be bubbling, indicating the existence of a bronchial fistula. In addition, the cystic formation in the upper lobe was communicating with that in the lower lobe. They mainly concerned the dorsal segment of the upper lobe, the apical segment of the lower lobe and the medial segment of the middle lobe. These findings argue in favour of MAKP of the lung involving all three lobes.

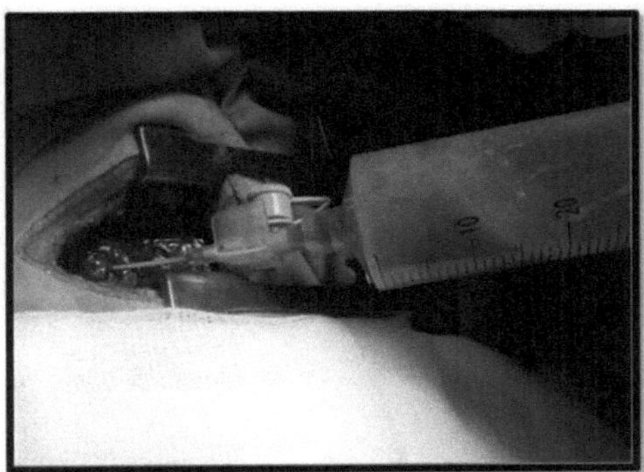

Figure 42. Pus-producing cystic formation.

Rather than perform a right pneumonectomy, we decided to perform an atypical resection of each of these 3 cystic formations. The latter did not have their own wall, which led us to perform a pericystectomy, removing the cyst and the necrotic tissue adhering to it. During this pericystectomy, other pus-filled cystic formations were discovered. This pericystectomy was total in the periphery and partial in depth because of the risk of damaging the bronchi and lobar arteries.A post-operative chest X-ray showed the disappearance of the pulmonary opacity and the absence of pleural effusion **(Fig. 43)**.

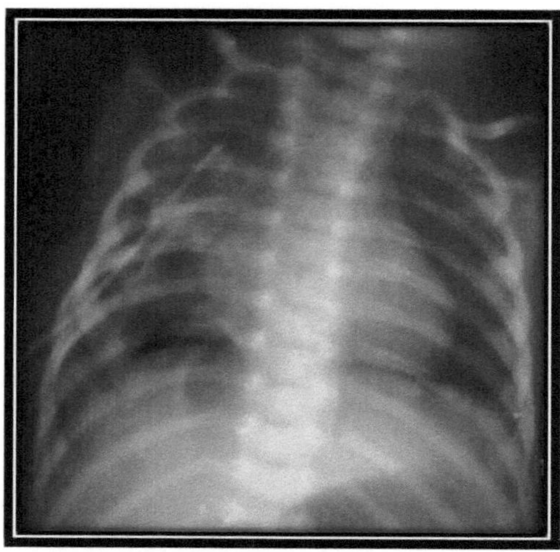

Figure 43. Post-operative radiological check: disappearance of the pulmonary opacity.

Histological examination of the surgical specimens showed that the samples were made up of unrecognisable lung tissue due to severe inflammation. This inflammation affected the alveoli, which often had a cubic metaplasia of their epithelial lining with a lumen occupied by macrophages with foamy cytoplasm, sometimes associated with foreign body type giant cells. There were also areas of fibrosis and others where the lung parenchyma was filled by granulation tissue particularly rich in macrophages and neutrophils. This tissue sometimes surrounded cavities such as those seen around abscesses. There were no epithelioid granulomas or histological images suggesting an underlying pulmonary malformation. Anatomopathological examination concluded that **there was significant acute and chronic inflammation of the lung tissue.** The patient was lost to view.

COMMENT 11

The infant (T.I.) was female, 23 months old, with no particular pathological history, who presented at the age of 22 months with a respiratory symptom consisting of a hacking cough, dyspnoea and a fever of 39°C. Radiological examination revealed a cystic fluid formation in the right upper lobe, 3.8 cm in diameter, with a hydroaerobic level. Antibiotic treatment resulted in the development of an aerotic, right apical cystic formation with a regular wall and no hydroaerosic level, initially suggestive of right upper lobe PKA **(Fig. 44 a and b)**.

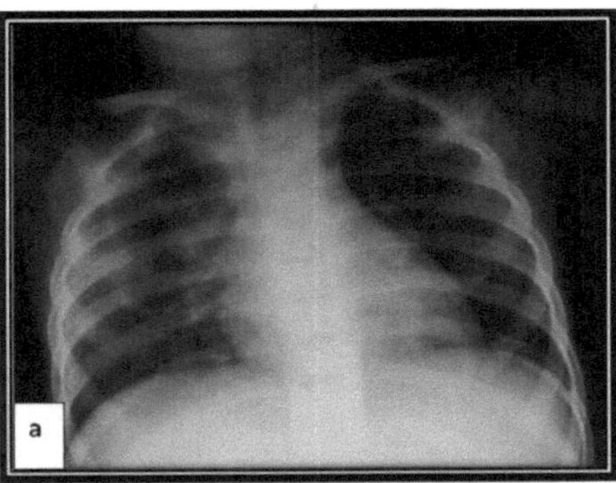

Figure 44 a. Front chest X-ray: regular-walled aerotic cystic formation in the right upper lobe.

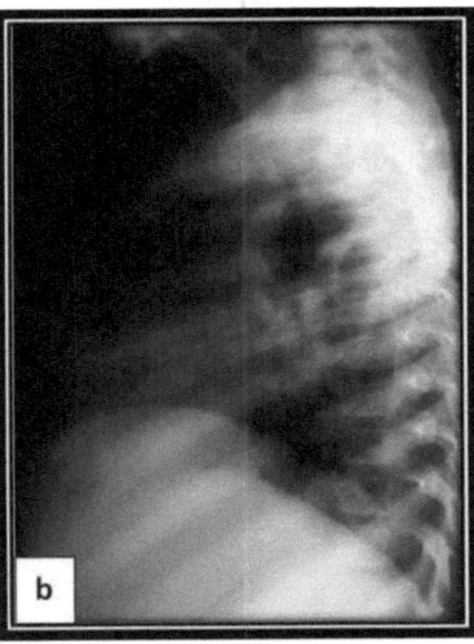

Figure 44 b. Profile chest X-ray: hyperclarity of the right upper lobe with posterior projection.

A thoracic CT scan ordered some time after the infectious episode confirmed the existence of an aerotic multi-cystic formation, measuring 3x1.5 cm, with a regular thickened wall and no hydro-aeric level **(Fig. 45)**.

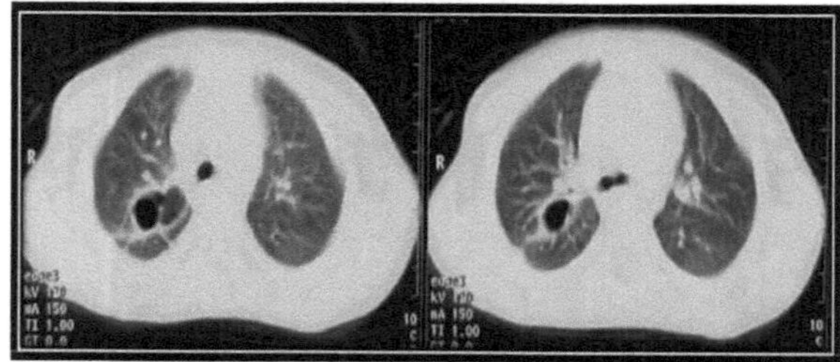

Figure 45. Chest CT: multi-cystic aerotic formation in the right upper lobe.

Bronchoscopy revealed no foreign body.

Given the recurrence of febrile bronchopneumonia, the complication o f purulent pleurisy and the persistence of the same parenchymal cystic images on radiological investigations, the diagnosis of right upper lobar MAKP was raised.A right posterolateral thoracotomy to the 5th intercostal space was performed. There were numerous very dense pleural adhesions in the upper lobe and the apical segment of the lower lobe and numerous mediastinal adenopathies. A right upper lobectomy was performed. Cefotaxime antibiotic prophylaxis was started. Post-operative care was straightforward and the infant was discharged to his parents after 5 days. Histology of the lobo-isthmectomy specimen **showed a focus o f inflammatory fibrous tissue.** However, there was no histological evidence of MAKP. The subsequent course was favourable with a 4.5-year follow-up. The chest X-ray was normal **(Fig. 46).**

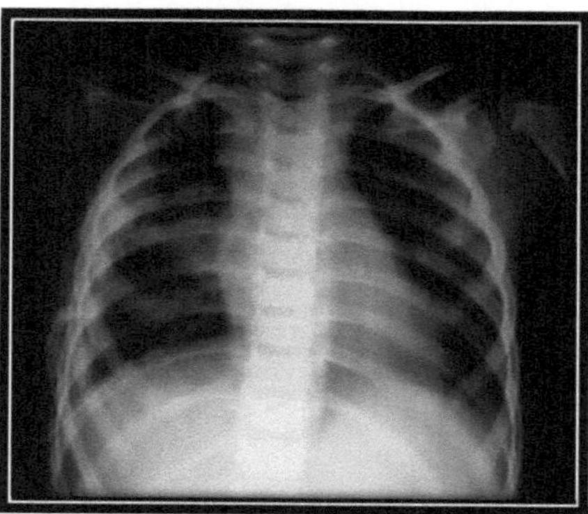

Figure 46. Radiograph chest of X-ray: good lung expansion.

COMMENT 12

The newborn baby (B.M.) was male, 22 days old, f r o m a poorly monitored pregnancy, with a history of hospitalisation at t h e   age of 5 days for polypnoea and expiratory whining associated with jaundice and refusal to feed. Given the positive history of infection, the diagnosis of maternal-foetal infection was raised, but the infectious work-up was negative. A chest X-ray was ordered, showing a right pneumothorax which recurred after 2 exsufflations. Physical examination revealed polypnoea at 54 cycles per minute. Pulmonary auscultation showed diminished vesicular murmurs on the right.The chest X-ray showed a complete right pneumothorax, compressive with deviation of the mediastinum to the left **(Fig. 47)**.

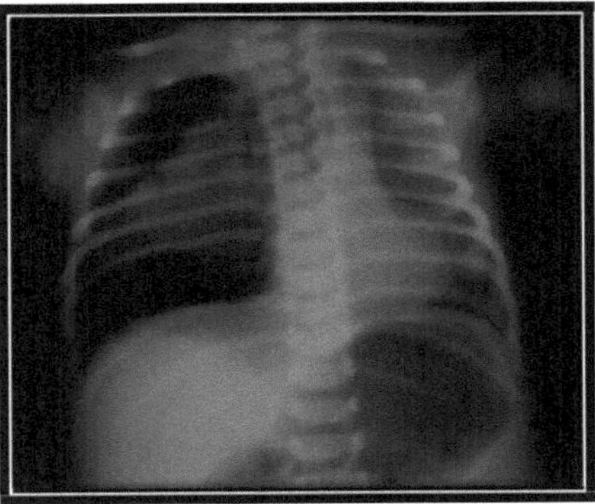

Figure 47. Chest X-ray: right total and compressive pneumothorax with deviation of the mediastinum to the left.

After exsufflation of the pneumothorax, the chest X-ray showed a well-limited homogeneous clearness 4 cm long, projecting from the lower third of the right lung field **(Fig. 48)**.

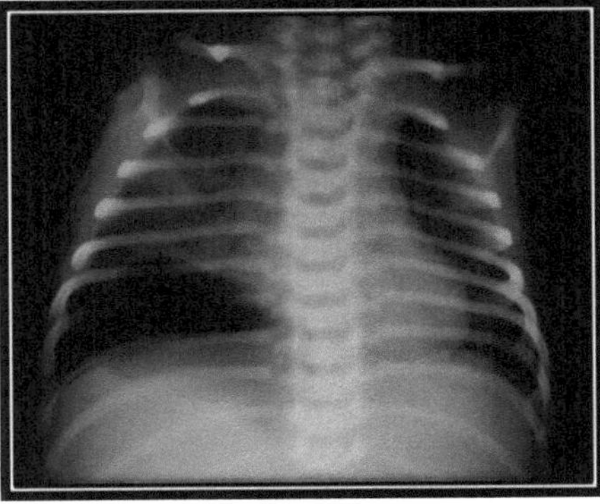

Figure 48. Chest X-ray after exsufflation: clarity of the right lower lobe.

Chest CT confirmed the existence of an air cystic mass in the right lower lobe. This formation had a clean, thickened wall and was 4 cm long.There was also an abundant right pneumothorax with the mediastinum displaced to the left. The right lung was collapsed **(Fig. 49)**.The diagnosis of right lower lobar MAKP was suspected and the newborn was scheduled for lobectomy. On examination, the right lower lobe was attached to the diaphragm by numerous fibro-inflammatory adhesions. There were no obvious abnormalities in the right lower lobe, The right middle and upper lobes were normal. Palpation of the right lower lobe showed that its entire diaphragmatic surface was covered with cardboard, and it was at this level that there were adhesions with the diaphragm.

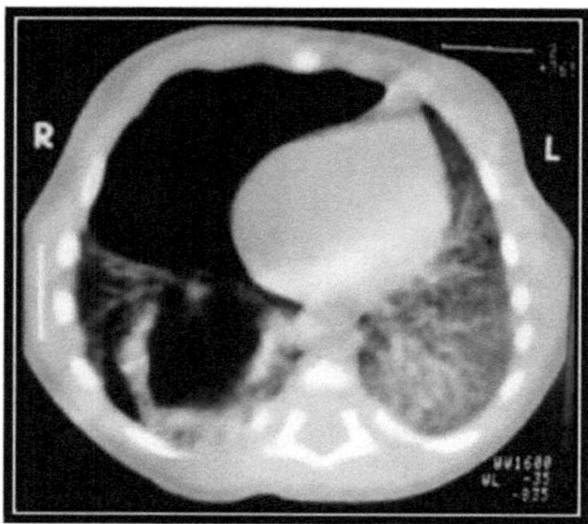

Figure 49. Chest CT scan: air cystic formation in the right lower lobe and right pneumothorax with deviation of the mediastinum to the left.

Since it was difficult to determine the exact location of the malformation by inspection and palpation, and since the thoracic CT scan could not give the exact location of the cyst, a right lower lobectomy was performed. Ampicillin antibiotic prophylaxis was instituted. The post-operative course was straightforward, with removal of the chest tube on the 3rd post-operative day.On cross-section, the lung parenchyma was condensed and fairly well vascularised. There was no macroscopically obvious cystic lesion. Histologically, the various samples examined had a similar appearance. The lung parenchyma showed no lesions. histological features **apart** from a **discrete distension alveolar in the peripheral lung.** The chest X-ray after 1 month showed good expansion of the right lung **(Fig. 50)**.

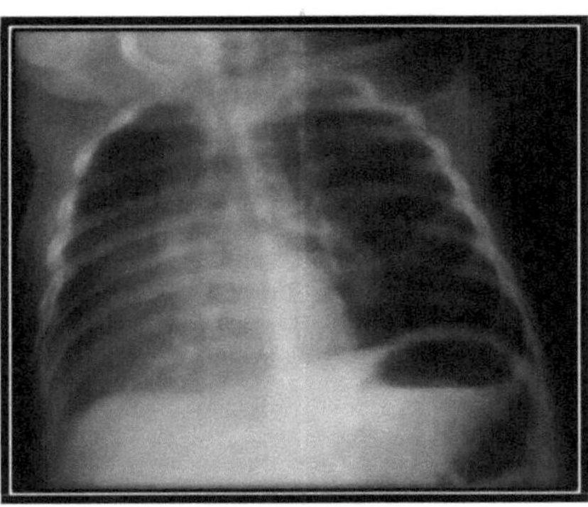

Figure 50: Chest X-ray: good expansion of the right lung.
The patient was subsequently lost to follow-up.

COMMENT 13

A 6-month-old female infant (B.M.) from a normal pregnancy, with a history of bronchoalveolitis treated as an outpatient with a good outcome, presented with cough and dyspnoea with fever one week prior to hospitalisation.

On pulmonary auscultation, the right vesicular murmurs were diminished. Biological tests showed a hyperleukocytosis of 11,700 per mm3 and a CRP of 34 mg.$^{ml-1}$. A chest X-ray was ordered, showing a voluminous excavated opacity with a hydro-aeric level occupying the entire right lung field. A supplemental thoracic CT scan revealed a voluminous, compartmentalised fluid collection in the right hemi thorax measuring 10x6x8 cm, with a clean wall that enhanced after injection of the contrast medium. This collection had a drainage bronchus (right lower lobar bronchus). It exerted a significant mass effect, pushing back the mediastinum and right lung parenchyma. It was associated with a ^{2nd} fluid cystic formation, homogeneous, unilocular, in the posterior mediastinum, with a thin wall measuring 3 cm in length **(Fig. 51)**.A radiographic check was carried out one day later, showing complete emptying of the hydroaerosic collection, which had been replaced by a voluminous clarity occupying the entire right lung field (Fig. 52).The infant was started on Cefotaxime-Teicoplanin and scheduled for surgery. Intraoperative exploration revealed a right lower lobe with a cystic formation, most probably related to macrocystic PKA.

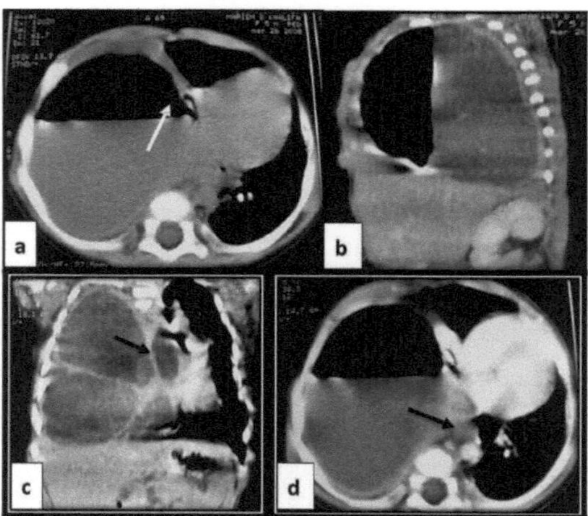

Figure 51. a and b: Chest CT: watery collection in the right hemi thorax with draining bronchus (arrow). **C and d:** Chest CT: posterior mediastinal cystic mass (arrow).

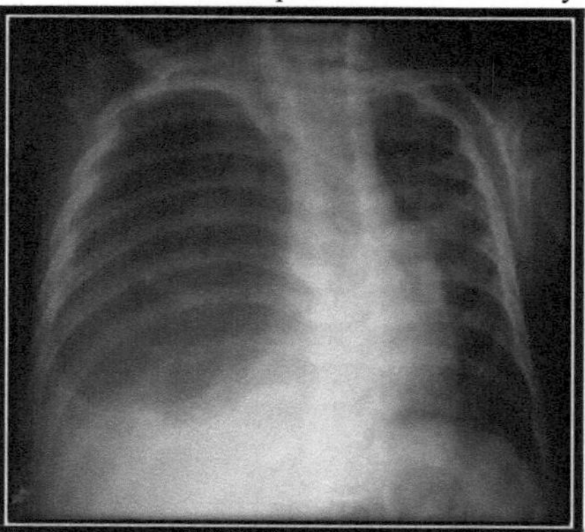

Figure 52. Chest X-ray: large right lung field.

In other cases, investigation revealed extra-lobar pulmonary sequestration and a bronchogenic cyst in the posterior mediastinum not communicating with the oesophagus. A right lower lobectomy, resection of the pulmonary sequestration and mediastinal bronchogenic cyst were **performed (Fig. 53).**

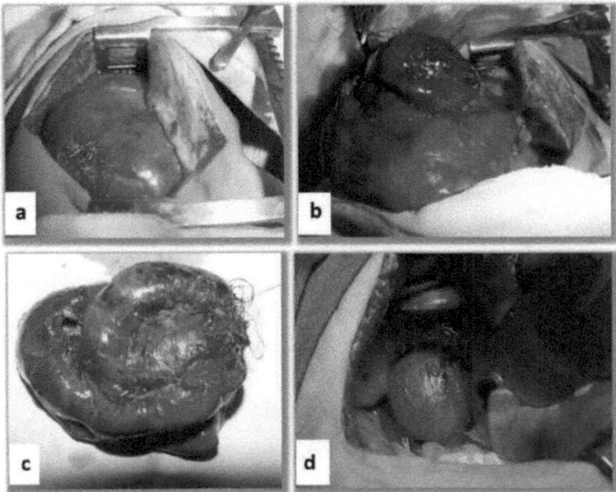

Figure 53. a and b: Intraoperative appearance. **c:** Lobectomy specimen for right lower lobar MAKP. **d:** Mediastinal bronchogenic cyst with extra-lobar sequestration.

Post-operative management was straightforward, with removal of the chest tube on day 11, and the infant was discharged to his parents the following day. The chest X-ray on discharge showed good lung expansion **(Fig. 54)**.

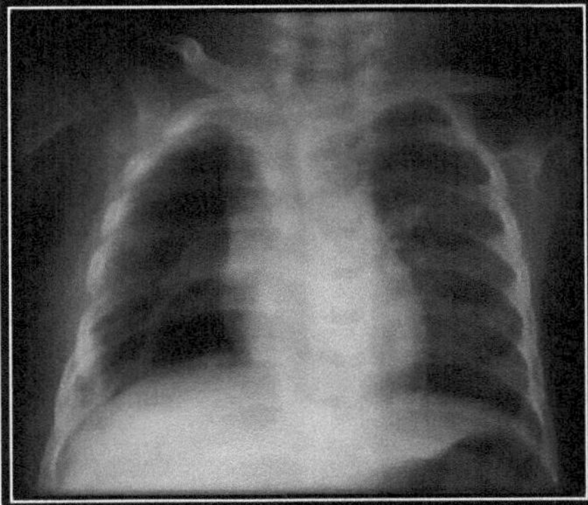

Figure 54. Check radiological control: good right pulmonary expansion.

Histologically, several samples were taken and showed that the wall of the cystic parenchymal formation was made up of fibrous tissue bordered by granulation tissue rich in neo-vessels and a polymorphic inflammatory infiltrate. In a single specimen, the cystic wall appeared to be lined with respiratory epithelium. This cystic formation could correspond either to **an encysted abscess** whose wall is partially epithelialised, probably as a result of its communication with a bronchiole, or to a **type I MAKP.** The mediastinal cyst corresponded **to a cyst of the primitive intestine.** Its wall was lined with epithelium of both respiratory and

39

squamous types. The rest of the wall resembled a digestive wall made up of a muscular mucosa, a sub-mucosa and a muscularis with its two internal and external layers.The third sample corresponded **to pulmonary sequestration.** The follow-up was 18 months. At the last clinical check-up, the patient was asymptomatic.

COMMENT 14

The daughter (S.H.), aged 3, presented with a productive cough, abdominal pain and fever, treated symptomatically with no improvement. On physical examination, the child was apyretic and eupneic.The biology revealed a hyper-leukocytosis of 18,000 per mm3, a sedimentation rate of 87 at 1 hour and a CRP of 50 mg.L-1. A hydatid serology test was carried out, which came back negative. The chest X-ray showed a cystic formation in the left lower lobe measuring 3 cm in major axis, with a hydroaerobic level **(Fig. 55)**.

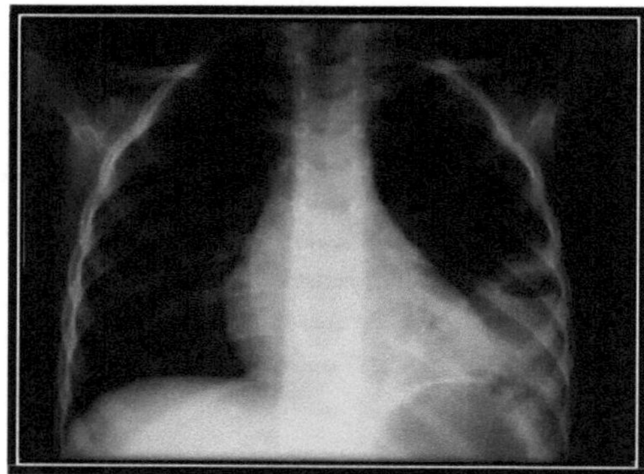

Figure 55. Front chest X-ray: left lower lobar hydroaerobic formation.

Thoracic ultrasound confirmed the presence of a left basal cystic lesion with homogeneous, thick contents and a thick wall. The thoracic CT scan showed systemic involvement of the anterior and lateral-basal segments of the left lower lobe with the presence of a formation of 4 cm in diameter (Fig. 56).

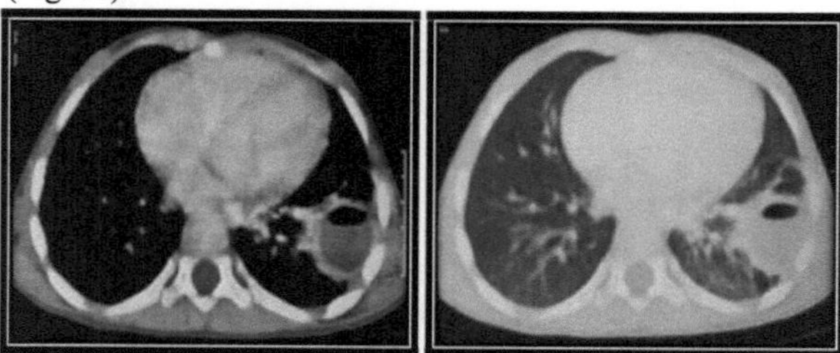

Figure 56. Chest CT scan: systemic involvement of the anterior and lateral-basal segments of the left lower lobe with the presence o f a hydroaerobic formation.

A chest X-ray showed the disappearance of the hydro- aeric level and the persistence of a blurred opacity with poor limits at the base of the left lung **(Fig. 57 a and b)**.

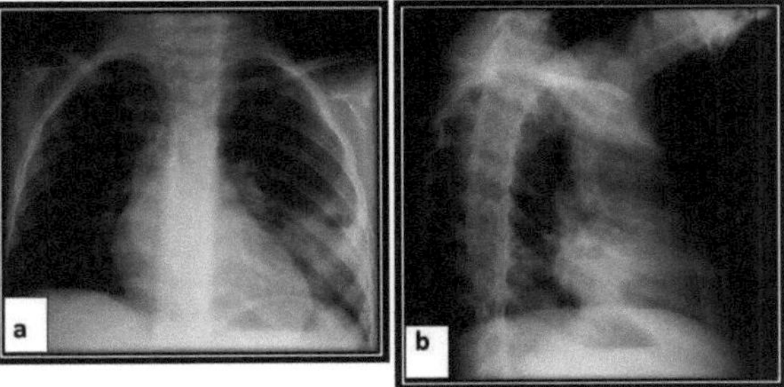

Figure 57. a: Control radiograph of the front chest: poorly defined opacity of the left basal lung. **b:** Radiograph of the side chest: blurred opacity of the left basal lung.

The girl underwent a posterolateral left thoracotomy to the 5th intercostal space. Intraoperative examination revealed numerous adhesions between the parietal pleura and a cystic formation in the left lower lobe involving the anterior and lateral-basal segments, measuring 2.5 cm. On opening, this formation was full of pus, which was removed for bacteriological examination. The rest of the lobe was normal **(Fig. 58)**.

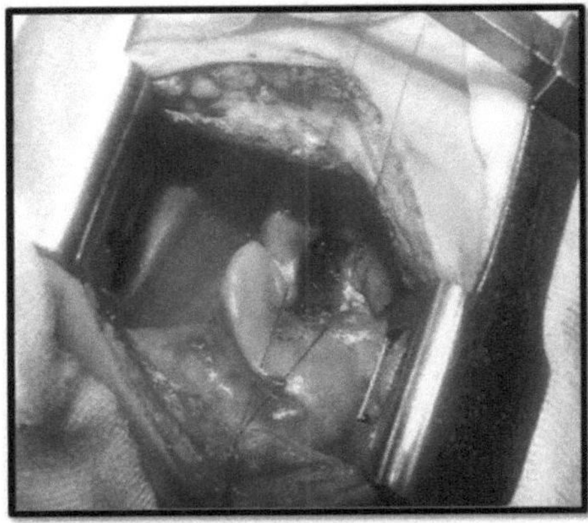

Figure 58. Intraoperative appearance suggestive of a lung abscess.

Given that the cyst did not exceed 2.5 cm in size and that the rest of the lower lobar parenchyma was normal, and in view of an appearance reminiscent of a lung abscess, rather than performing a lobectomy, we opted for complete removal of the peri-cyst. The post-operative course was straightforward.Histologically, the specimen involved the wall of a cyst, the inner surface of which was lined with respiratory-type epithelium that was often abraded. The rest of the wall was made up of connective tissue and smooth muscle with an inflammatory infiltrate rich in lymphocytes. This cystic wall was prolonged by lung tissue

41

showing dilated bronchioles filled with macrophages.In addition, there were lesions of vegetative alveolitis, characterised by the presence of loose connective tissue buds filling the alveolar lumen.The interstitial tissue contained a dense inflammatory infiltrate rich in lymphocytes that clustered together.In view of this histological appearance, it was concluded that the **patient had MAKP of the left lower lobe.**The follow-up was 10 years. The girl had no respiratory symptoms. Radiological examination revealed no parenchymal abnormalities and lung growth was normal.

CHAPTER III
RESULTS

Our series included 14 children (10 girls and 4 boys) aged between 23 days and 4 years. During the same period, 47 patients underwent surgery for histologically confirmed MAKP. The percentage of diagnostic and therapeutic errors in our series was (14/61) 29, 78%. This figure can be explained by the attitude of the surgeon in the face of the "simple doubt" of MAKP and the persistence of fever in the face of a unilocular cystic lesion.

1. History and Diagnosis antenatal
No family history of bronchopulmonary malformation was reported. No case benefited from antenatal diagnosis.

2. Symptomatology clinical
The age of onset of symptoms ranged from 1 day to 3 years. These were:

- Neonatal respiratory distress in 3 cases (cases 1, 2 and 12).

- Recurrent bronchopneumonia in 2 cases (cases 4 and 6).

- Febrile pleuropneumonia not improved by antibiotic treatment in 7 cases (cases 3, 7, 8, 9, 11, 13 and 14).
- Haemoptysis in 1 case (case 5).

Elsewhere, it was a chance discovery in 1 case (case N°10).

3. Biology
A biological inflammatory syndrome was noted in 6 cases (cases N°7, 8, 9, 10, 11 and 14). A tuberculin TST and a test for Kokh's bacillus in the sputum were requested for case 5 and were negative. Hydatid serology was requested in 2 cases (cases N°5 and 14) and came back negative.

4. Radiology

⬥ **Chest X-rays** were taken in all patients:

- Air cystic images in 2 cases (cases 1 and 2).

- A clear cystic image in 3 cases (cases 3, 4, 12).

- A hydro-aeric formation in 5 cases (cases N°7, 8, 11, 13).

- A water-toned opacity in 3 cases (cases 6, 9 and 10).

- Alveolar opacity in 2 cases (cases 5 and 14).

Chest CT scans were performed in all patients.

The diagnosis of MAKP was suspected in 13 cases. It showed:

- Air cystic images in 4 cases (cases 1, 2, 6 and 10).

- Air cystic formation in 4 cases (cases 3, 4, 11 and 12).

- A hydro-aeric formation in 4 cases (cases N° 7, 8, 9 and 13).

- Images of parenchymal condensation in 1 case (case 5).

In 1 case (case 14), the thoracic CT scan showed systematised involvement with the presence of a rounded hydroaerobic formation, raising the suspicion of lung abscess.

Thoracic Doppler ultrasound in 3 cases (cases 2, 5 and 14) did not show any systemic vessels vascularising the malformation.

The TOGD performed in 2 cases showed massive gastro-oesophageal reflux in 1 case (case N°4).

5. Lung perfusion scintigraphy

Performed only on case 1, it revealed hypoperfusion of the right upper lobe.

6. Endoscopy

The bronchoscopy requested in 1 case (case N°11) did not reveal any foreign body.

7. Associated malformations

Cardiac ultrasound in 1 child (case 6) was normal. No patient underwent karyotyping.

8. Available at

All children were treated surgically by posterolateral thoracotomy. The surgical procedure consisted of a lobectomy removing the malformation in 11 cases, a bi-lobectomy in 1 case (case N°1) and atypical removal of the cystic formations in 2 cases (cases N°10 and 14). The malformation involved the lower lobe in 8 cases (cases N°2, 4, 5, 6, 7, 12, 13 and 14), the upper lobe in 4 cases (cases N°3, 8, 9 and 11), the upper and middle lobes in 1 case (case N°1), and the right pulmonary field in 1 case (case N°10).

9. Evolution

Post-operative management was straightforward in 12 cases. Microcytic hypochromic anaemia requiring transfusion was observed in 1 case (case 1). One infant died immediately post-operatively following a nosocomial infection (case N°6). The chest tube was removed between the 2nd and 11th postoperative day. The hospital stay ranged from 5 days to 27 days.

The follow-up ranged from 1 month to 10 years. 2 children continued to have recurrent bronchopneumonia (case N° 1 and 4) until the age of 1 year and 30 months, respectively. 7 patients were lost to follow-up (cases N°3, 7, 8, 9, 10, 12 and 13).

10. Anatomopathological study of the surgical specimen

The anatomopathological study of the surgical specimen was carried out in all cases and rectified the diagnosis in all 14 cases, concluding with:

- Pulmonary interstitial emphysema in 1 case (case 1).

- An antenatal pulmonary infarction in 1 case (case N°2).

- Neonatal pulmonary infarction in 1 case (case 3).

- Postnatal pulmonary infarction in 1 case (case 4).

- Bronchial dilatation lesions secondary to a plant foreign body in 1 case (case 5).
- Capillary pulmonary haemangiomatosis in 1 case (case 6).

- Lung abscess in 4 cases (cases 7, 8, 9 and 10).

- Acute and chronic inflammation of the lung in 1 case (case N°11).

- Alveolar distension without MAKP lesions in 1 case (case 12).

- A hybrid lesion combining MAKP type I, a cyst of the primary intestine and pulmonary sequestration in 1 case (case N°13).
- MAKP of the left lower lobe treated by partial resection rather than lobectomy (case 14).

1. Definition

MAKP or "Craig's disease" is a segmental hamartomatous lesion of the lung. It results from an arrest in the maturation of the conduction pathways in the bronchioles without the formation of alveolar tissue. It was first described in 1897 by Staerk [8, 9] and individualised by Ch'in and Tang in 1949 [10, 11]. It is defined as an adenomatoid proliferation of the terminal respiratory structures, manifested by cysts bordered by cylindrical or cubic epithelium [6, 12].

2. Aspect macroscopic

The affected lobe is enlarged, dense and heavy. It has a firm consistency and a smooth, pinkish surface. On sectioning, cystic cavities vary in number and size [6, 13] (Fig. 59).

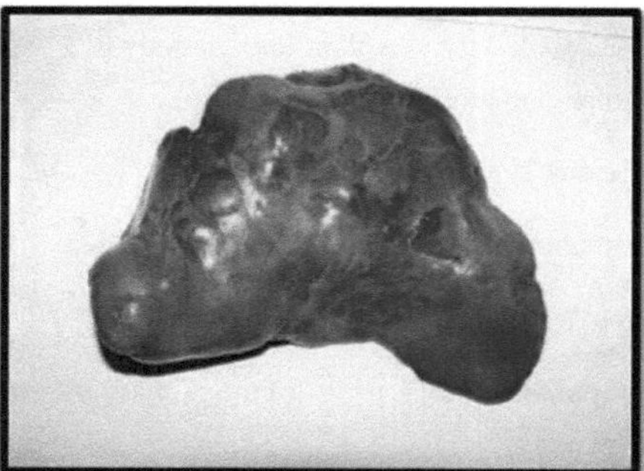

Figure 59. Macroscopic appearance of a lobectomy specimen for MAKP (enlarged lobe with multiple cysts).

There are communications between the cysts and between these cysts and the bronchial tract. These connections can form valve systems, allowing fluid to be evacuated during airborne life, with the development of air cysts which are often increasingly voluminous [13]. The blood supply is bronchial. A voluminous systemic artery is sometimes visible. It may disappear during the last trimester of pregnancy [13, 14].

3. Histological aspect

Only histological study confirms the diagnosis and eliminates other cystic pulmonary malformations [6]. In 1962, Kwitken and Reiner [6] described basic histological criteria for differentiating MAKP from other types of congenital cystic lung disease:

i. Adenomatoid appearance of the terminal respiratory structures forming communicating cysts of variable size covered with pseudostratified cubic and ciliated epithelium;
ii. Polypoid appearance of the mucosa with focal increase in elastic tissue in the cyst wall, beneath the bronchial epithelium;
iii.Absence of cartilage in the cystic parenchyma (except as a normal component of an adjacent bronchus, sometimes trapped within the lesion);
iv.Mucous cells grouped together on portions of the cyst wall or in the form of glands near pseudoalveolar structures;
v. Occasional presence of mucinous-lined alveoli;

vi.Absence of inflammation [6, 13].

These histological features may be associated with inflammatory phenomena attributable to superinfections [6].

4. Epidemiology

4.1. Age

Almost all cases of MAKP are diagnosed during the first two years of life. Sporadic cases have been reported in adulthood [6, 13]. In our series, the age at diagnosis of lung lesions ranged from 23 days to 4 years.

4.2. Gender

MAKP affects both sexes equally [1, 15]. A slight male predominance has been reported [6, 15].In our series, there was a predominance of females, with 10 girls and 4 boys.

5. History

N o racial or genetic predisposition has been reported, although familial cases have been described [5, 6]. In our series, no history of bronchopulmonary malformation was reported.

6. Incidence

It is difficult to establish because a BPCM may remain asymptomatic and unrecognised. MAKP accounts for approximately 25% of bronchopulmonary malformations [4, 5, 6, 12].Its incidence is 1 case per 25,000 to 35,000 births [2, 12, 16]. The advent of antenatal ultrasound has enabled early diagnosis of MAKP, allowing neonatal management [5, 6, 17, 18]. MAKP is the the bronchopulmonary malformation most frequently diagnosed antenatally [4, 5, 19].

7. Location

MAKP is often unilateral [2], generally affecting the lower lobes. Both lungs are affected with the same frequency [20]. Tropism of the right lung has been reported [6]. Extension to several lobes may occur [12, 13] and bilateral involvement is extremely rare [6]. In our series, the right-hand side is the most affected.

8. Classifications

8.1. Stocker classification [4, 5, 6, 12].

It is based on macroscopic aspects, histological criteria and the presence or absence of associated congenital malformations [6]:

➥ **Type I** (50%): Multiple cysts greater than 2 cm in diameter or a single large cyst with surrounding small cysts containing air and/or fluid **(Fig. 60)**. This type has the best prognosis.

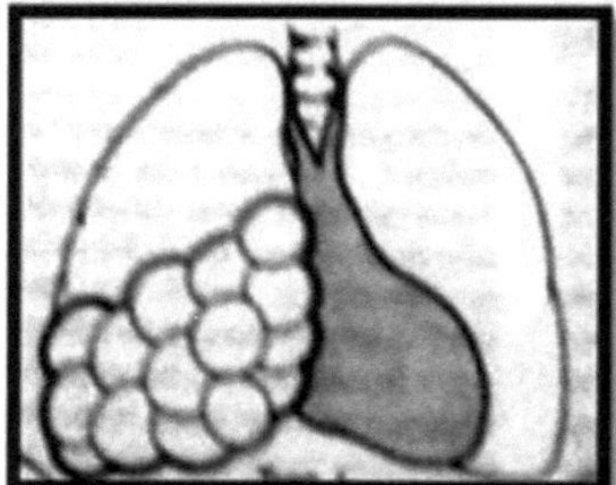
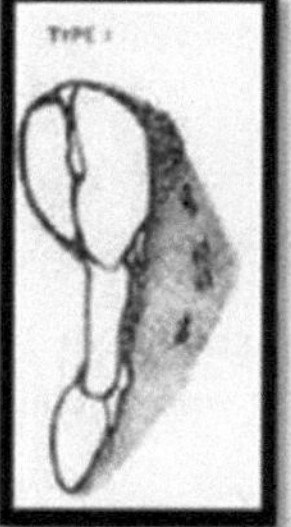

Figure 60: Aspect of a Stocker type I MAKP.

➥ **Type II** (40%): Multiple cysts less than 1 cm in size **(Fig. 61)** associated in 70% of cases with other congenital anomalies, particularly urogenital.

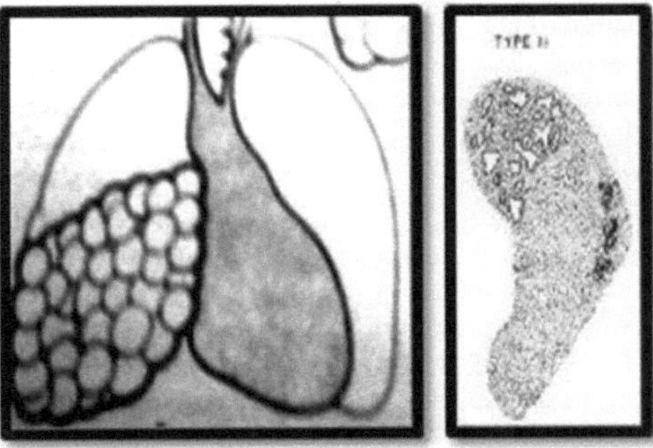

Figure 61. Aspect of a Stocker type II MAKP.

➕ **Type III** (10%): Small cysts less than 0.5 cm in diameter presenting as a solid mass **(Fig. 62)**. It represents the worst prognosis.

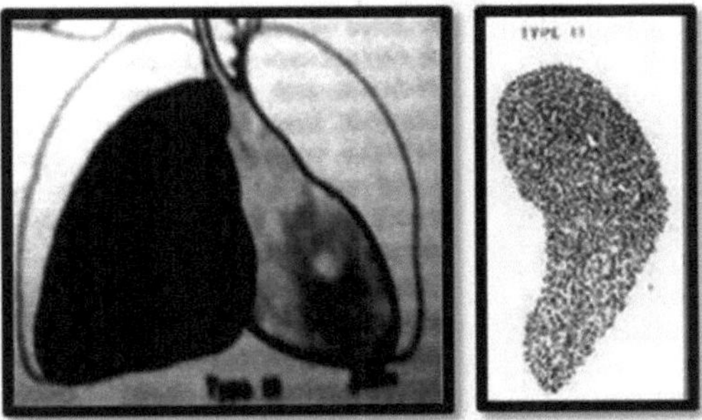

Figure 62. Aspect of a Stocker type III MAKP.

However, this classification is imperfect because it is purely histological and does not correspond to the pathophysiological mechanisms identified as being different **[21]**. Furthermore, it was established on post-natal data and seems less and less appropriate for describing lesions observed in the foetus. Numerous intermediate aspects are observed, and prognostic factors are poorly related to this summary description **[21]**. The classification has now been completed and MAKP has been extended to congenital malformation of the pulmonary tract, divided into 5 histological types according to the size of the cysts and their histological resemblance to the bronchial and aerial structures (Tab. I) **[1, 12, 23]**.

Table I: Classification of congenital malformations of the pulmonary tract [12].

Type/ Topography	Features macroscopic	Features microscopic	Age at diagnosis, prognosis	Frequency
0:tracheobronchial	Diffuse involvement of the five lobes	Cysts less than 0.5 cm in diameter, bordered by pseudostratified ciliated epithelium Vessels far from these structures making the gas exchange impossible	Death at birth	<2%
1:distal bronchi, proximal bronchioles	Large cysts 2 to 10 cm in diameter	Cysts lined with pseudostratified ciliated epithelium Wall containing smooth muscle and elastic tissue Normal adjacent alveoli	Until adulthood	60 à 70%
2: bronchioles	Multiple small cysts 0.5 to 2 cm in diameter	Small cysts lined with ciliated columnar or cuboid epithelium, sometimes containing elastic tissue and a fibrotic barrier. muscular	Neonatal Poor prognosis Accompanied by other malformations	10 à 15%
3: distal bronchioles/ alveoli	Cysts smaller than 0.5, often affecting several lobes Dense, mass-like appearance	Mixture of cysts and solid tissue, adenomatoid proliferation of acinar origin Cysts lined with non-ciliated cuboid epithelium	Neonatal Poor prognosis	5 à 10%
4: acinar	Large cysts	Large cysts lined of pneumocytes I and II	Neonatal and childhood Associated with blastoma pleuropulmonary	10 à15%

8.2. Adzick classification

A second classification introduced by Adzick is simpler and above all more clinical, based on anatomical, ultrasound and prognostic criteria. It describes 2 types of PKA: macrocystic and microcystic **(Tab. II)** [14, 23, 24, 25].

Table II: Classification of MAKP according to Adzick

Type	Ultrasound appearance	Prevalence
Macrocystic	One or more cysts :? 5 mm in diameter, anechoic within tissue that is more echogenic than healthy lung, of good prognosis	58%
Microcystic	Cysts < 5 mm in size, pseudosolid, often associated with hydrops, with a poor prognosis	42%

9. Clinical presentation antenatal

MAKP is most often diagnosed during t h e ultrasound scan in the fifth month of pregnancy [2, 26, 27].The sonographic appearance of these malformations is cystic, hyper-echogenic or mixed [2, 16, 20]. The antenatal hyper-echogenic appearance is not predictive of the histological diagnosis and may correspond to all other pulmonary malformations [2, 26]. In antenatal care, an ultrasound classification is used to distinguish micro-cystic forms (53%) from macro-cystic forms (22%) or mixed forms (25%) **(Fig. 63) [16]**.Antenatal ultrasound can be used to assess whether pulmonary involvement is isolated or not, to demonstrate systemic vascularisation using Doppler, to look for complications, to establish a prognosis and to set up follow-up in order to optimise peri-natal management [2, 26]. Lesion associations should be sought, in particular with extra-lobar pulmonary sequestration and bronchial atresia, for example, which once again draws attention to the embryo-pathological proximity of these lesions [23].

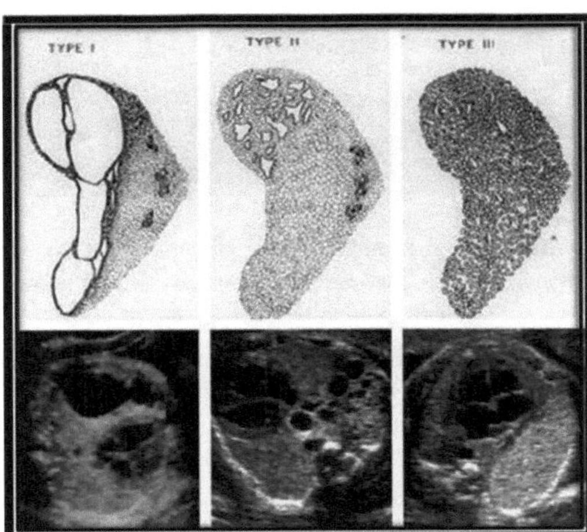

Figure 63. MAKP, correlation of histological appearance with antenatal ultrasound appearance.

In Doppler mode, the vascularisation of the lesion is derived from the pulmonary vascularisation, with normal spectra overall, but heterogeneous mapping suggestive of a dysplastic pulmonary lesion. The origin of the vascularisation of a hyper-echogenic intra-pulmonary lesion can be documented in all cases. In colour or energy mapping, a significant difference in the intensity of the vascularisation of the lesion compared with that of the healthy lung is suggestive of an evolving lesion **(Fig. 64) [23]**.

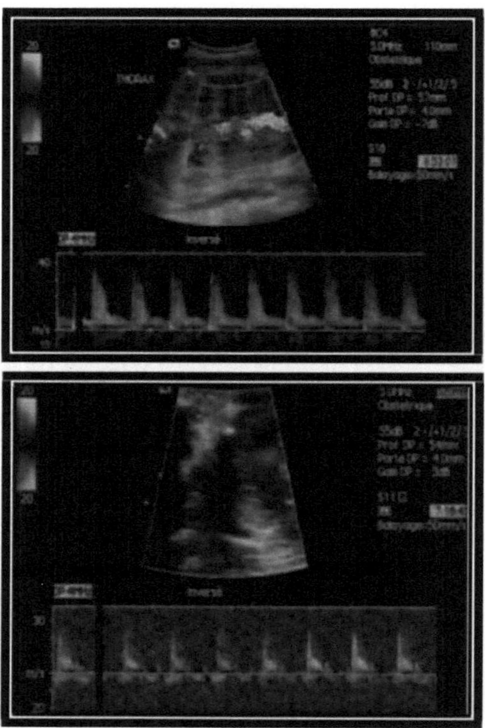

Figure 64. Recording of 2 types of spectra (systemic and pulmonary type) within the lesion of an associated form (MAKP and pulmonary sequestration).

Fetal magnetic resonance imaging (MRI) provides little additional information compared with ultrasound. Macrocystic forms appear as a heterogeneous hyperintense lobulated mass without feeder vessels, while microcystic forms appear as a homogeneous lobulated mass. Mediastinal displacement is also visible **[16]**. In our series, no case benefited from antenatal diagnosis.

10. Circumstances of discovery at postnatal

10.1. In the neonatal period

A meta-analysis shows that 80% of patients are asymptomatic during the neonatal period [2]. Follow-up of asymptomatic patients at birth includes a standard chest X-ray, taken before discharge from t h e maternity hospital. This may appear normal even if there is a persistent lesion. Chest CT scans are generally performed in the first two to three months o f life in asymptomatic patients [2]. Twenty per cent of patients ae symptomatic at birth. Neonatal respiratory distress is the most common complication [2, 5, 20, 27]. In the absence of surgical treatment, around 3% of patients develop symptoms at a median age of seven months. Pulmonary infections are the most common complication beyond the neonatal period [2, 20]. Other complications include pneumothorax and haemothorax. Pneumothorax is rare, however, and should be investigated for pleuropneumoblastoma.In rare cases, MAKP may remain asymptomatic and be discovered by chance [6].

10.2. More later

MAKP can also be diagnosed in children or even adults in the presence of cough and recurrent pulmonary infections, which are peculiar in that they always affect the same area [7, 20], with the eventual formation of abscessed masses due to inadequate alveolar drainage [6].

In most patients, MAKP is suspected on the basis of clinical criteria and radiological images [2, 6]. The patient has a persistent or recurrent non-productive cough, with a mono-lobar multi-locular cystic mass, a hydro- aeric level, and no vascular abnormalities. The clinical picture is multifaceted, and the problem is to always be aware of it in the event of recurrent pulmonary infections in order to ensure appropriate management and avoid potential infectious or neoplastic complications [6].

11. Radiological aspects

11.1. Standard radiography

For many authors, chest X-rays from the front and the side are the first-line complementary examinations sufficient to establish the diagnosis of bronchopulmonary malformations [5, 15].False positives and negatives have been described. In the post-natal period, the chest X-ray may show a more or less homogeneous opacity which gradually becomes aerated, with the appearance o f one or more cystic lesions of variable size depending on the histological type [1, 4, 7].

MAKP may be responsible for a large, hyper-clear lung if the walls are thin, imperceptible on standard radiology **(Fig. 65)**. It may be responsible for a mass effect on adjacent structures, in particular displacement of the mediastinum to the contralateral side [1, 7]. In our series, a chest X-ray performed in all patients suggested the diagnosis of MAKP in 13 cases. It showed cystic aeritic images in 2 cases, a clear cystic image in 4 cases, a hydro-aeric formation in 3 cases, a watery opacity in 3 cases and an alveolar opacity in 1 case.

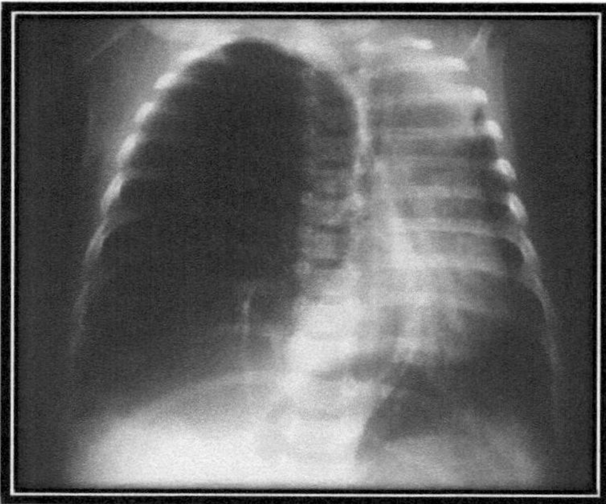

Figure 65. Front chest X-ray: right lung over-distended, hyper-clear with deviation of the mediastinum to the left in relation to MAKP of the right lower lobe.

11.2. Thoracic ultrasound and Doppler

Thoracic ultrasound is of little use in the post-natal period. It can differentiate between the liquid and solid nature o f a bronchopulmonary malformation. Similarly, it can rule out a diaphragmatic hernia by demonstrating digestive images in the thorax [28]. Combined with colour Doppler, it can point to pulmonary sequestration by showing an aberrant aortic artery feeding the malformation [4].In our series, thoracic Doppler ultrasonography performed in 3 cases did not show any systemic vessel vascularising the malformation.

11.3. CT scan thoracic

This examination helps to confirm the diagnosis suspected on the chest x-ray, assess the extent of the lesion and its anatomical relationships with the tracheobronchial tree and vessels [1, 29], rule out a differential diagnosis and discuss treatment, particularly in terms of size and impact on the healthy parenchyma [2, 4, 5]. The radiological appearance depends on the type of malformation and whether or not there is a complication. In macrocystic forms (types 1 and 2), the lesions a r e well-demarcated, thin-walled aerial cystic structures, with at least one lesion larger than 20 mm in type 1 and lesions of uniform size, measuring between 5 and 20 mm in type 2 **(Fig. 66) [1]**.

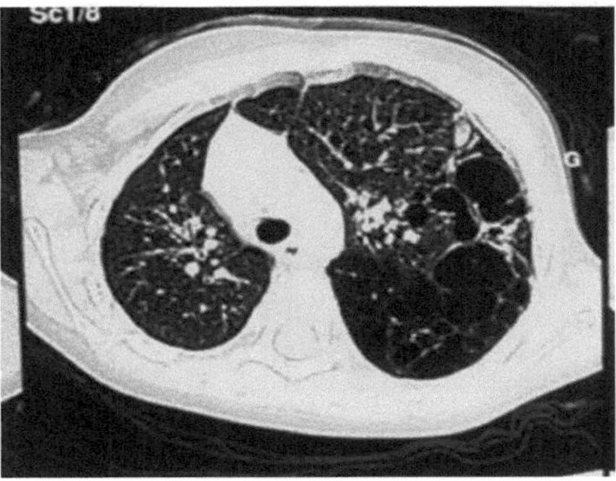

Figure 66. Chest CT scan: MAKP type 2 of the left lung.

The density of lung tissue at the contact point is variable, with the possibility o f ventilation problems (atelectasis).In type 3, the microcysts are indistinguishable and form a heterogeneous mass of condensation with ill-defined contours. Type 4, which usually appears as large cysts, cannot b e distinguished from a cystic form of grade I pleuropulmonary blastoma [1].Systemic arterial vascularisation may be associated in 30% of cases and should be systematically sought, particularly in type 2 patients [1, 2, 31]. Helical CT and angioscanner are therefore indicated to highlight vessels 1mm in diameter and to better assess the lung parenchyma and abnormalities of the bronchial tree [7, 30]. The presence of thickened walls, enhanced after injection of contrast and/or a hydroaerobic level may indicate infection. Pneumothorax is a rare but potentially life-threatening complication [1, 4]. In our series, chest CT scans were performed in all patients. The diagnosis of MAKP was suspected in 13 cases. It showed air cystic images in 4 cases, an aeriform cystic formation in 4 cases, a hydro-aeriform formation in 4 cases and images of parenchymal condensation in 1 case.

12. Other examinations

12.1. MRI thoracic

It is of little value in this pathology and is only used in the event of diagnostic difficulties. It analyses the content of the malformation and specifies its extension **(Fig. 67) [4, 6]**.

12.2. Lung perfusion and ventilation scintigraphy

It delineates the extent of the functional territory in relation to the pathological territory [32]. Lung perfusion and ventilation scintigraphy is particularly useful for making a differential diagnosis with congenital lobar emphysema [33].

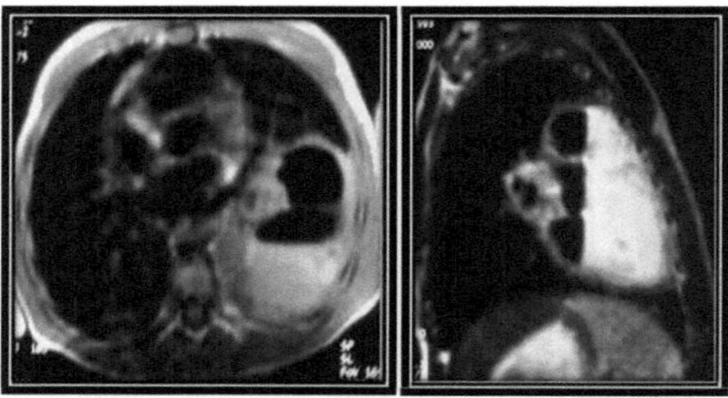

Figure 67. Thoracic MRI: large multi-locular cystic lesion, left lower lobar.

13. Diagnostic problems

They arise as early as antenatal diagnosis, in view of the variable appearance on antenatal ultrasound. False negatives may be due to the small size of the lesion or to technical difficulties inherent in the reduction of acoustic windows associated with costal mineralisation (especially during the third trimester) [20]. The post-natal radiological differential diagnosis is that of circumscribed hyper-clarity [6].

13.1. Congenital hernia of the diaphragmatic cupolas

It is due to a defect in closure of the pleuroperitoneal duct occurring between the 8th and 10th week of gestation [34, 35, 36]. Antenatal ultrasound may show anechoic intra-thoracic images corresponding to digestive structures, absence of lung tissue on the same side, deviation of mediastinal structures and absence of integrity of the diaphragm. Hydramnios occurs in half of all cases [37]. This initial ultrasound assessment is supplemented by fetal MRI data, which can be used to assess not only the morphology but also the volume and a certain degree of functionality of the lungs [38]. MRI can be used to differentiate MAKP from congenital herniation of the diaphragmatic cupolas, which can be difficult to detect on ultrasound [28, 39]. Study of the signal allows better characterisation of the intra-thoracic organs, which is particularly interesting in cases of diaphragmatic hernia. In T1, the liver appears in relative hyper-signal and the colonic framework is in frank hyper-signal; in T2, the stomach and small intestines appear in hyper-signal (Fig. **68)** [40].

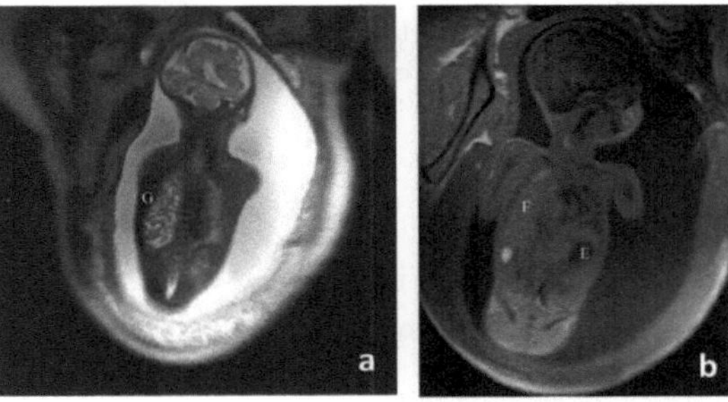

Figure 68. Right diaphragmatic hernia on T2 (a) and T1 (b) weighted sequences.

In the post-natal phase, misdiagnosis is common due to the absence of typical symptoms. There are two clinical pictures of very different severity:

• Early respiratory distress occurring immediately or within a few hours of birth. The earlier the symptoms, the greater the pulmonary dysplasia and the poorer t h e prognosis.

• The late presentation occurs a few days or months after birth and is characterised by respiratory signs (dyspnoea, cough, repeated bronchopulmonary infections, etc) or digestive signs (vomiting, abdominal pain, occlusive syndrome, etc) [41, 42].

Diagnosis is essentially based o n careful examination of the chest X-ray, which should never be ruled out if it is previously normal.

The radiological appearance is polymorphous and depends on the anatomical type of hernia, and the radiological image is variable due to the intermittent nature of the hernia.

The chest X-ray may show:

• A heterogeneous opacity or hydroaeric images occupying one half of the thorax with effacement of the diaphragmatic dome on that side.

• A deviation of the mediastinum towards the contralateral side **(Fig. 69)** [43].

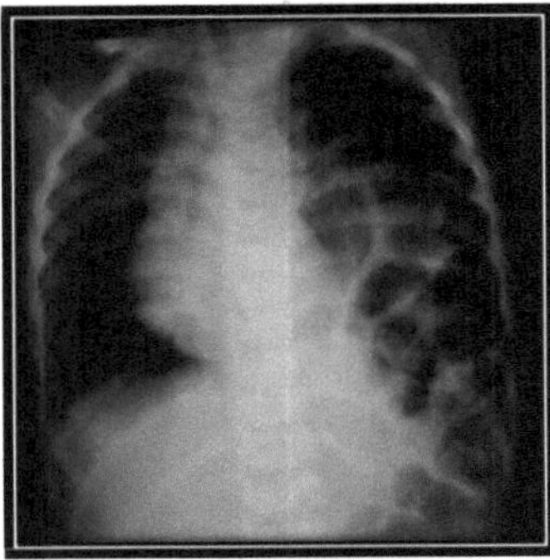

Figure 69: Front chest X-ray: intra-thoracic digestive tract lesions.

Upper opacifications are requested first and foremost in non-emergency cases, in the presence of basi-thoracic hydro-aerosic images, thus enabling the position of the stomach and the first coves to be determined [42, 43].

Thoraco-abdominal ultrasound may show:

• A solution for the continuity of the dome.

• Digestive tracts in t h e hemithorax, following their course from the abdomen.

• Echogenic images belonging to the spleen or the left lobe of the liver.

A multi-slice CT scan with multi-planar reconstructions enables a precise diagnosis of the thoracic images and confirms the presence of a herniated orifice, its size and the nature of the herniated organs **(Fig. 70)**.

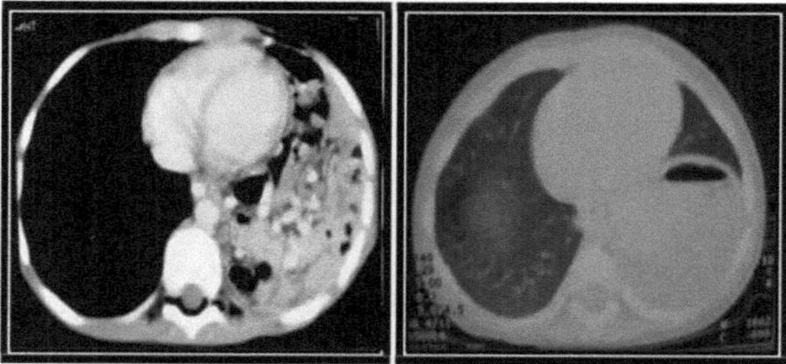

Figure 70. Thoracic CT scan: digestive structures in the left intrathoracic region.

MRI may sometimes be performed to rule out other malformations when the standard radiological appearance and opacification are not conclusive [43]. Treatment is surgical and consists of closing the diaphragmatic defect [44].

13.2. Sequestration lung

It's a condition rare which represents 0.15 à 6.5% of malformations pulmonary arteries [4, 45]. It is defined as an area of non-functional lung tissue, characterised by disconnection from the bronchial and vascular structures and vascularisation by one or more systemic arteries originating either directly from the thoracic or abdominal aorta, or from one of its collaterals [45, 46].It occurs in 98% of cases in the lower lobes [4]. There are two types of pulmonary sequestration: intra- and extra-lobar (Tab. III).

Table III. Intra- and extra-lobar pulmonary sequestration.

Intra-lobar sequestration: 75%.	Extra-lobar sequestration: 25
Common pleural envelope	Clean pleural envelope
Systemic arterial pedicle	Systemic arterial pedicle
Pulmonary venous return	Systemic venous return

Antenatal diagnosis is possible using foetal ultrasound and MRI. Doppler ultrasound is able to visualise more specifically the image of an aberrant artery arising from the aorta, but also the sequestration itself in the form of a more or less well-limited echogenic solid mass, sometimes the site of cystic images **(Fig. 71)**. Doppler ultrasound can sometimes be used to visualise venous drainage **[47, 48]**.On fetal MRI, lung sequestration appears hyper-signal on T2-weighted sequences and hypo-signal on T1-weighted sequences **[39]**. The circumstances in which pulmonary sequestration is discovered vary widely.While extra-lobar sequestrations are most often asymptomatic, and can therefore be discovered radiologically or surgically, intra-lobar sequestrations may be revealed by episodes of haemoptysis, isolated chest pain, pleurisy, but above all on the occasion of recurrent pulmonary infections with fever **[45]**. However, some cases of sequestration may be discovered following spontaneous haemothorax or heart failure due to a major shunt. Clinical examination is often normal apart from complications **[46]**.

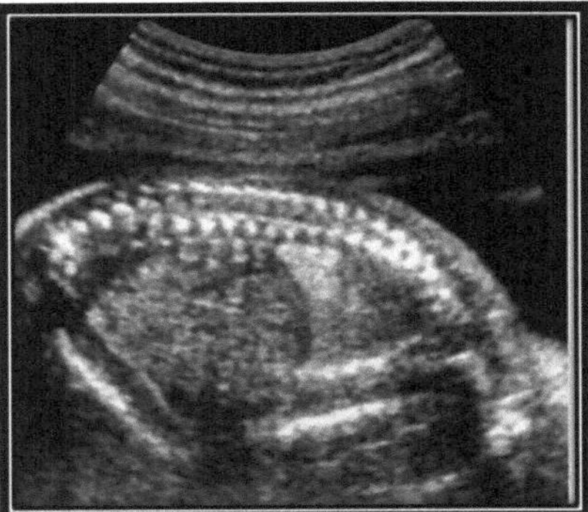

Figure 71. Pre-natal ultrasound showing a very suggestive aspect of sequestration in the form of a triangular, left basal, juxta-diaphragmatic, hyper-echogenic image.

Associated malformations are not uncommon. They may include diaphragmatic hernia, MAKP, bronchogenic cyst **[49]**, communication with the oesophagus and stomach, digestive duplication and diverticulum, vertebral, cardiovascular or genitourinary anomalies **[45]**. The most classic radiological appearance is that of an opacity most often located in the postero-basal segment of the lower lobe.In the event of infection or communication with the airways, the sequestration takes on a polycystic appearance combining clear and dense areas and sometimes liquid levels [45, 46, 48].A clear, thick-walled bulla-like image is rare. It should be discussedMAKP, congenital lobar emphysema or bronchogenic cyst [49, 50]. This radiograph may be normal in some cases of extra-lobar sequestration (Fig. 72) [46].

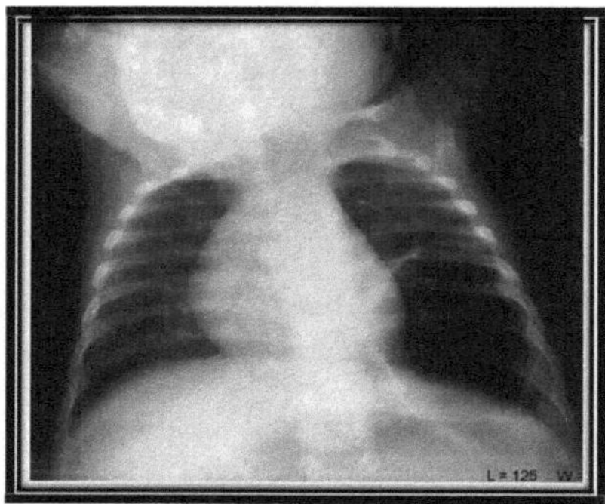

Figure 72. Front chest X-ray: bullous image of the left base surrounded by a thick wall.

Thoracoabdominal ultrasound can be used to visualise the mass and possibly identify the systemic artery when combined with Doppler.Thoracic CT allows the topography of the lesion and its nature to be better defined. Injection of contrast medium results in moderate and heterogeneous enhancement of the sequestration and visualisation of the systemic artery in 70% of cases **(Fig. 73) [45]**.

MRI, and in particular angio-MRI, is undoubtedly the ideal method for diagnosing pulmonary sequestration. It allows the lung mass to be visualised, its location to be determined and its relationship with the pulmonary, pleural and hilar structures. MRI angiography shows the systemic artery and venous return, and helps to clarify their relationship with the heart chambers **[46, 48, 51]**.

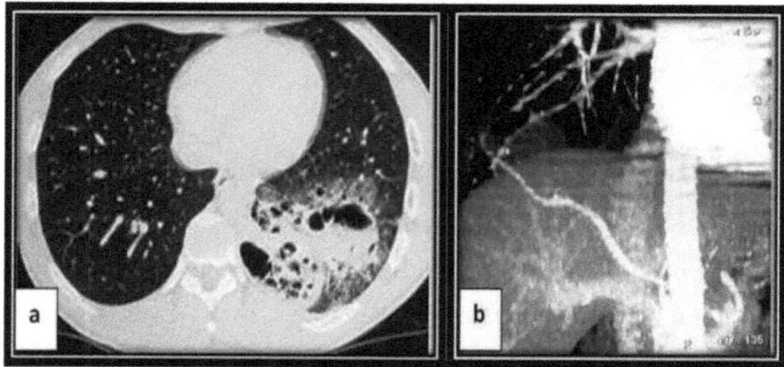

Figure 73. a: Parenchymal CT scan showing cystic intra-lobar sequestration in the left lower lobe. **B:** Reconstruction showing a small-calibre artery arising from the celiac trunk in a patient with intra-lobar sequestration of the right lower lobe. Venous drainage into the inferior pulmonary vein is also visible.

Pulmonary sequestration is treated surgically. This involves lobectomy in the case of intra-lobar sequestration and excisional surgery in the case of extra-lobar sequestration with ligation of the systemic vessels [46, 52]. Endo-vascular techniques are proposed for the treatment of pulmonary sequestration, essentially in children whose general condition is impaired or in patients with heart failure. This technique may be inadequate, in which case it must be supplemented by surgery [51]. The diagnosis is confirmed histologically: the sequestration appears macroscopically as a pinkish or yellowish mass with no anthracosis and a clear boundary with the neighbouring, normally aerated segment. The parenchyma is often atelectatic or dystrophic (Fig. 74) [53]. Microscopically, the sequestrum consists of several cavities with either a bronchial structure or a collagenous wall lined with cylindrical or flattened epithelium. The arteries are elastic. Areas of atelectasis or alveolar dysplasia may be noted (Fig. 75) [46, 51].

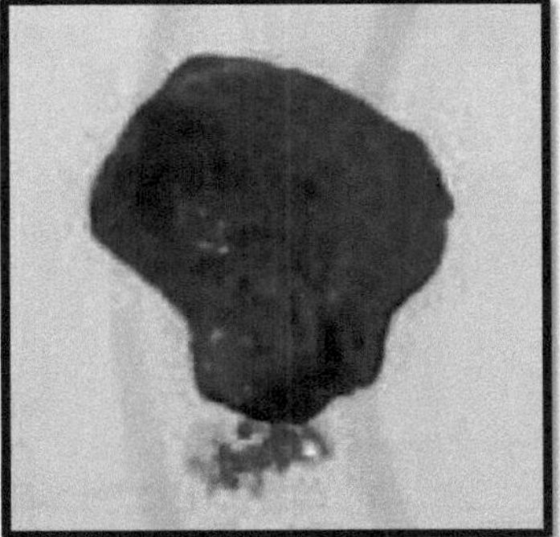

Figure 74. Surgical specimen of extra-lobar sequestration.

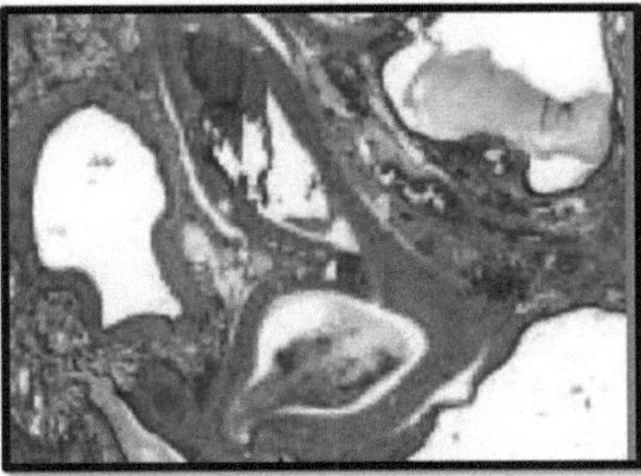

Figure 75. Histological appearance of pulmonary sequestration.

In our series, only observation N°13 represented a case of extra-lobar sequestration discovered per-operatively and forming part of a mixed malformation.

13.3. Congenital lobar emphysema

This is an abnormality of lung development characterised by a distension of a lung lobe without destruction of the parenchyma.Its prevalence, lower than that of MAKP, is thought to be around one in 50,000 pregnancies. It affects boys three times more often than girls. The left upper lobe is most often involved [4]. Congenital lobar emphysema is rarely described antenatally because non-specific ultrasound signs more often suggest MAKP [54, 55]. Its antenatal diagnosis is based on the observation of a hyper-echogenic pulmonary territory with a deviation of the mediastinum **(Fig. 76)**. This pulmonary hyper-echogenicity is not specific, making positive diagnosis difficult [33].

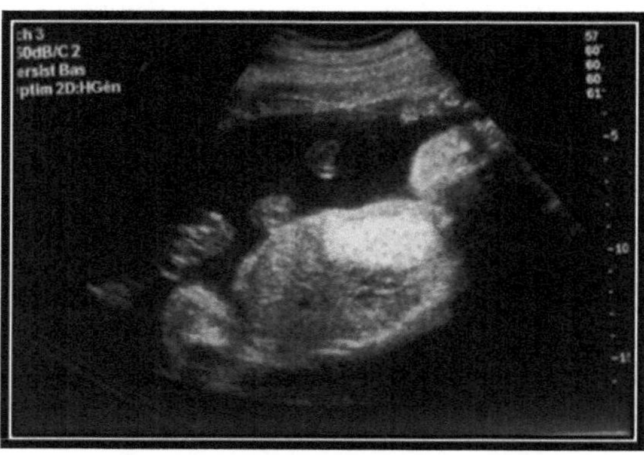

Figure 76. Antenatal ultrasound: hyper-echogenic lung and backward displacement of the heart.

Progressive attenuation of ultrasound signs is common, and may even disappear completely in the third trimester. The association of cystic pulmonary images is rare. This raises the problem of differential diagnosis between congenital pulmonary emphysema and MAKP. While the preferred topography of congenital pulmonary emphysema is upper and middle lobar, that of MAKP is lower and middle lobar. MAKP is essentially inferior lobar. Fetal MRI provides a good volumetric assessment of the lung lesion and an accurate evaluation of the healthy parenchyma, but a differential diagnosis is rarely possible [33]. The neonatal manifestations of congenital lobar emphysema (tachypnoea, cyanosis, respiratory distress) are variable and progressive in onset. The lesion is sometimes asymptomatic before revealing itself several weeks later, making systematic post-natal investigation of congenital lobar emphysema advisable, even when it is small in volume [56].

Chest X-rays and CT scans carried out in the post-natal period often enable a distinction to be made between congenital pulmonary emphysema and MAKP. The chest X-ray shows lobar distension in the form of hyper-clarity with trans-mediastinal herniation and displacement of the contralateral lung. There are also signs of thoracic distension. CT is more sensitive than X-ray in demonstrating distension and the small appearance of stretched and small vascular structures. It helps to localise emphysema, to search for a possible aetiology and to distinguish emphysema from other lesions. The CT scan of emphysema shows a hyperclarity associated with a trans-mediastinal hernia and a backflow of the mediastinum towards the contralateral side **(Fig. 77) [57]**.

Ventilation scintigraphy shows a decrease in ventilation of the affected lobe, which takes the form of a gap on inspiration and an isolated radioactive focus on expiration. Perfusion scintigraphy shows a perfusion defect **[56, 57, 58]**. Treatment consists of lobectomy. Surgical abstention is possible for asymptomatic or pauci-symptomatic lesions. However, because of the risk o f recurrent bronchopulmonary infections, some authors recommend systematic lobectomy **[59, 60]**.After surgical treatment, the evolution is favourable, with growth of the remaining lung reaching up to 90% **[61]**. The diagnosis of certainty can be made by histology of the specimen. operation which reveals the lesions of congenital emphysema **[33]**.

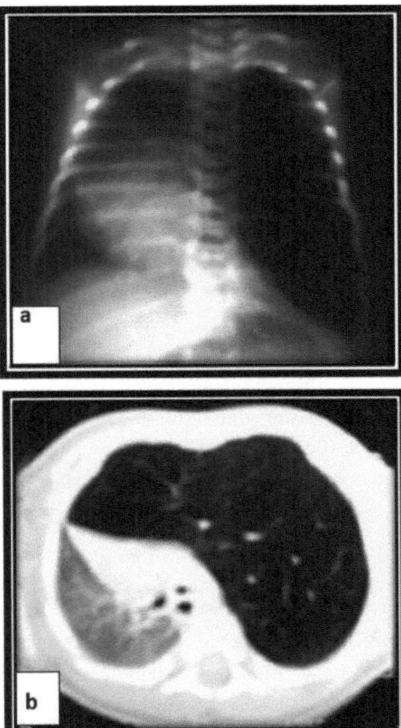

Figure 77. a: Chest X-ray: left lung hyperclarity and contralateral mediastinal deviation. **B:** Chest CT scan: left upper lobar emphysema.

13.4. Bronchogenic cyst

It is a benign cystic congenital tumour of bronchial origin occurring between the 3rd and 4th week of embryonic development. It is defined by its wall composed of a mucociliated respiratory epithelium secreting mucus, which is the source of the thick liquid content, frequently associated with other bronchial structures such as cartilage or respiratory glands [62, 63].Most bronchogenic cysts (75 to 85%) are located in the mediastinum along the tracheobronchial tree (para-tracheal, subcarinal, hilar, para-oesophageal or rarely in the oesophageal wall itself) [64, 65], but they may also be found in the lung parenchyma. Intrapulmonary cysts account for 15 to 25% of cases and are most often found in the peri-hilar regions or, rarely, in the peripheral lung, with a predilection for the lower lobes. Bronchogenic cysts only communicate with the tracheobronchial tree when they are infected [66].In antenatal care, intraparenchymal cysts can pose a diagnostic problem with MAKP on MRI. It corresponds to an intraparenchymal cyst, uni or sometimes multilocular, homogeneous, well limited and with a high signal in T2 weighting. MRI eliminates a solid formation if the contents are echogenic. It can help to distinguish it from a MAKP, in the case of air trapping [39].

Post-natally, the clinical presentation varies according to its size and location: respiratory distress in the newborn or infant, dyspnoea with stridor, atelectasis, haemoptysis, dragging pneumonitis, chest pain [62, 63]. There are also forms of the disease which have long been asymptomatic or even symptomless [62].

On chest X-ray and CT scan, the cyst appears as a well-defined, rounded mass with a fluid content. It may have a thin, regular, well-defined wall, which is easier to delineate with contrast injection. When there is communication between the cyst and the tracheobronchial tree, a hydroaerosic level is produced [66]. MRI is the examination of choice, allowing detailed analysis of the walls, contents and immediate environment of the cyst [62]. Surgical removal is the usual treatment for bronchogenic cysts. If excision is incomplete, excision of the mucosa is recommended. However, the diagnosis of certainty remains the anatomopathological examination: bronchogenic cysts are generally uniloculated. The cyst wall consists of fibrous connective tissue containing one or more components of the bronchial tree, such as smooth muscle, elastic tissue, cartilage, bronchial glands and nerve branches. This wall is lined with ciliated columnar epithelium, occasionally squamous [62, 67].

13.5. Interstitial pulmonary emphysema

This is a rare condition [68]. It is a classic complication of mechanical ventilation in premature newborns, occurring most often following the use of high ventilatory pressures, particularly in cases of hyaline membrane disease [69].

Some publications have reported the occurrence of pulmonary interstitial emphysema without any mechanical ventilation in term neonates [70, 71]. The pathophysiology was first described by Macklin in 1944 [72]. This emphysema is characterised by dissection of the pulmonary interstitium by air, resulting in rupture of the alveolar basement membrane, which allows air to pass through. This can occur following the aspiration of foreign bodies from the bronchi and bronchioles in neonates [70, 72]. The result is an accumulation of air in the pulmonary interstitium.

A distinction is made between:

• Acute interstitial emphysema.

• Persistent interstitial emphysema localised to one lobe.

• Persistent interstitial emphysema affecting the entire lung parenchyma
[73].

13.5.1. Acute interstitial emphysema

The passage of air from the interstitium to the adjacent spaces can lead to pneumothorax, pneumomediastinum or pneumopericardium. It is less frequently associated with mechanical ventilation and may occur spontaneously.

13.5.2. Persistent interstitial emphysema

The air persists within the interstitium [68].

13.5.3. Diffuse persistent pulmonary emphysema

It is often associated with bronchopulmonary dysplasia. Its prognosis is poor [68]. Diagnosis is suspected on thoracic CT scan: diffuse interstitial emphysema appears as small cysts varying in size from 0.2 to 3 mm in diameter. 0.5 cm [74]. The management of newborns with diffuse persistent pulmonary emphysema depends on the severity of respiratcry distress. Treatment may be conservative or more aggressive, involving pneumonectomy. The conservative approach includes simple measures such as lateral decubitus positioning and selective obstruction or intubation on the side of the emphysema. Early surgical intervention should be undertaken in neonates with progressive disease, and segmentectomies or lobectomies of the most affected lobe are preferable to pneumonectomies. Localised persistent interstitial emphysema is rarer. It may occur spontaneously or be associated with hyaline membrane disease.A bronchial fibroscopy, when feasible, may be indicated to look for an obstacle (granuloma, bronchomalacia, etc) which may be curable [69].

Localised interstitial emphysema appears on chest X-ray as a uni or multilocular aerotic cystic formation. It may be predominantly unilateral, leading in severe forms to displacement of the airways. compression of the contralateral lung which becomes atelectatic (**Fig. 78**). Chest CT can be useful in differentiating it from other cystic air lesions in the lung, such as MAKP or congenital lobar emphysema.

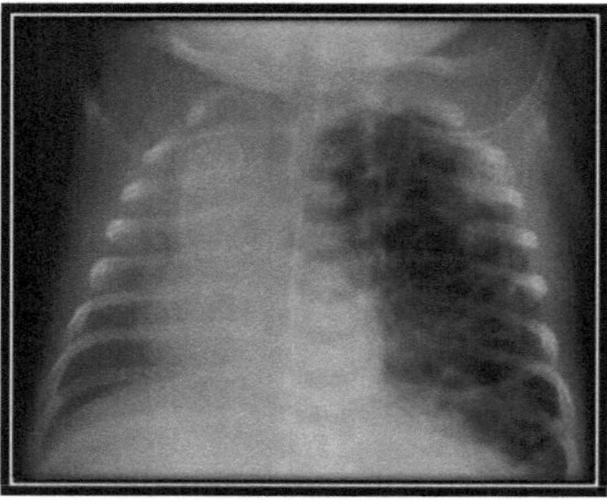

Figure 78. Front chest X-ray: multiple cystic aeri involving the left lung.

Interstitial emphysema lesions do not respect the normal pulmonary architecture, which is dissected by the cysts, with centrilobular and paraspinal involvement. The cysts are separated by thin partitions. There is often a deviation of the mediastinal elements towards the contralateral side and a trans-mediastinal hernia **(Fig.79)**.

In favour of MAKP:

• The presence of lesions in the neonatal period.

• The cysts are larger and more variable in size.

• The usual association with a nodular or pseudo-tissue component [68].

It is essential to distinguish interstitial emphysema from other cystic bronchopulmonary diseases because treatment may be non-operative **[73]**.

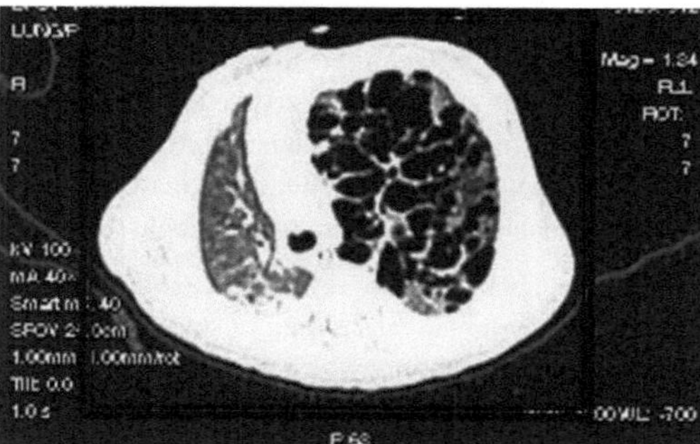

Figure 79. Chest CT scan: appearance of interstitial emphysema localised to the left lung: multiple cysts of varying size dissecting the interstitial tissue.

Various management techniques have been recommended:

• Simple measures: saline washes with selective aspirations, lateral decubitus positioning to the side of the emphysema.

• A course of corticosteroids lasting a few days is sometimes suggested to relieve local inflammatory obstruction.

• In severe cases resistant to these measures, selective ventilation of the contralateral lung may be used, either by selective intubation or by obstruction using a balloon catheter on the side of the emphysema.

Selective intubation is easy on the right, but technically difficult and delicate on the left, and can be poorly tolerated.

Obstruction on the emphysematous side is better tolerated. It can be relieved by regular intervals (every 2 to 4 hours) to allow aspiration. T h e effectiveness of selective obstruction appears to be closely linked to the state of the lung parenchyma [69].

• High frequency oscillation ventilation (HFO) is an alternative that has been proposed for interstitial emphysema [75].

• Resection of the affected lobe may be indicated if there are signs of pulmonary compression by large cysts, atelectasis, persistent respiratory distress or recurrent infections.

All in all, treatment is mainly preventive, and conservative treatment should remain the approach of choice. Pathological examination reveals multiple optically empty cystic cavities of variable size. These cavities are located in the septa separating the lobules. The cyst wall is made up of one or two layers of cells. The mucosa contains connective tissue with single-nucleated cells. The presence of multi-nucleated giant cells is pathognomonic. Our review of the literature reported 30 cases of pulmonary interstitial emphysema, 2 of which were treated as MAKP [75, 76]. In our series, we report 1 case of diagnostic and therapeutic error.

13.6. Bronchiectasis or dilatation of the bronchi

They are defined by permanent and irreducible dilatation of the bronchi associated with impairment of their function in more or less extensive areas [66].

There are 2 types:

• Diffuse form: affecting both lungs to varying degrees as the disease progresses. The conditions involved are immune and mucociliary clearance deficiencies.

• Localised form: affecting a segment or a lobe. In this case, the bronchiectatic lesions frequently affect the middle lobe and the lingula. This form may follow bronchial obstruction by stenosis or a foreign body, as in our case N°5 (a plant foreign body) [77].

There are many circumstances in which it may be discovered, and the first symptoms appear in the majority of cases at pre-school age [78].

Chest X-rays and CT scans are the key diagnostic tests, preferably carried out after preparation with long-term antibiotic therapy and respiratory physiotherapy. On CT, bronchiectasis is characterised by an enlargement of the internal bronchial diameter compared with the satellite artery (increase in the broncho-arterial ratio), the absence of narrowing of the bronchial lumen towards the periphery and the visualisation of bronchi less than 1 cm from the costal pleura. These signs are often associated with bronchial parietal thickening. Cystic bronchiectasis most often appears as clusters of aerated spaces, of heterogeneous distribution, adjacent to the corresponding pulmonary arteries, which may contain hydro-aerobic levels related to the accumulation of secretions in their declinal portions. Their walls may be thin or thick, with thickening indicating inflammation [79]. Bronchiectasis can be difficult to diagnose with MAKP when there is peripheral parenchymal hyperclarity associated with air trapping. Lung perfusion scintigraphy is easy to perform and highly sensitive, and its functional study provides essential information to complement the results of CT scans. The combination of lung perfusion scintigraphy and CT scan highlights the extent of the lesions and helps determine the choice between medical treatment and surgery. The use of single-photon emission computed tomography coupled with CT would facilitate the management of these patients, with savings in terms of cost, dosimetry and radiation protection [80]. Treatment of bronchiectasis is based on antibiotic therapy in the event of exacerbation in diffuse forms, and surgical removal is indicated in the following cases symptomatic and localised forms. Respiratory physiotherapy is always indicated [81].On pathological examination, the air space represents the dilated bronchi. The bronchial wall is the site of an inflammatory infiltrate and oedema during exacerbation phases. In chronic forms, the bronchial glands may be hyperplastic, and the bronchial wall is thickened and replaced by granulation tissue and fibroblastic proliferation. The ciliated columnar epithelium is often replaced by squamous metaplastic epithelium [66].

13.7. Ante and post natal pulmonary infarction cysts

This entity was first described by Stocker in 1987 [82]. Some authors suggest that occlusion of the main pulmonary artery may be responsible for the formation of pulmonary cysts [83]. It may occur before or after birth.Ischaemic necrosis of the lung parenchyma within a haemorrhagic zone is observed. Subsequently, fibrosis develops, transforming the infarct into a scar. The location of the cyst is peripheral, sub pleural, often on the right, as in 2 of the 3 cases in our series.The post-natal form often occurs in older children and young adults. Pre-natal onset explains the cases seen in newborns [83]. The association with heart disease such as persistent ductus arteriosus and atrial septal defect has been reported. Chest X-rays and CT scans reveal an aerotic cystic image, which is often uni-locular. Post pulmonary infarction cysts can be complicated by pneumothorax in older children. Histologically, there is a subpleural cystic formation within necrotic material, with a thickened, sparsely cellular wall, devoid of epithelial coating. The presence of keratin lamellae indicates ante-natal involvement. The lung tissue around the lesion may contain thrombosed arteries. Our review of the literature identified only 5 cases of post pulmonary infarction cysts in children [82, 83, 84]. Our series reports 3 cases of pulmonary infarction, 1 of which was ante-natal.

13.8. Capillary haemangiomatosis lung

This is a rare condition, characterised by diffuse or localised capillary proliferation that may infiltrate vascular, bronchial and interstitial structures, and may be responsible for pre-capillary pulmonary hypertension [85, 86, 87, 88]. It was first described by Wagenvoort in 1978 [88]. Very few data are available from patients with histologically confirmed capillary pulmonary haemangiomatosis. Almogro et al [89] pooled data from 35 cases of pulmonary capillary haemangiomatosis in the literature [86, 89].The pathogenesis of pulmonary capillary haemangiomatosis is still unknown. One proposed theory is that adaptation to hypoxia causes vascular changes and angioproliferation. Folkman and Klagsbrun [quoted by 88] described a group of angiogenic diseases (retinopathies, infantile haemangiomas, angiofibomas, psoriasis) characterised by a proliferation of normal capillaries attributed, for several authors, to a hypoxia-sensitive factor; the Vascular Endothelial Growth Factor (VEGF). Other authors consider the disease to be a hamartomatous lesion or a low-grade vascular tumour [88]. Familial forms with autosomal recessive transmission have been described [88]. Pulmonary capillary haemangiomatosis is most often discovered in adulthood, exceptionally in childhood after the age of 6, in the presence of secondary signs of pulmonary arterial hypertension (dyspnoea, haemoptysis and right heart failure). It is exceptional in newborns and infants and should be suspected in the presence of neonatal respiratory distress associated with pulmonary hypertension, cardiomegaly and bi-ventricular hypertrophy [88, 90]. The association with dilated cardiomyopathy and renal and bladder agenesis has been reported [88]. In the literature, there have been 3 paediatric cases of capillary pulmonary haemangiomatosis, including 2 neonates and 1 infant aged 11 months [88, 90]. The case in our series was aged 3 months. Biological tests are of little help, and associated thrombocytopenia has been reported [91]. Chest X-rays show poorly defined reticulo-nodular opacities with no specificity [92]. Cardiac Doppler ultrasound is useful for studying the impact of pulmonary arterial hypertension on the heart chambers [93]. Chest CT may show Kerley B lines or pleural effusions when pulmonary oedema occurs. Apart from this characteristic situation, it may show centro-lobular ground-glass opacities, septal lines and mediastinal adenopathies [94]. Thoracoscopic lung biopsies are of great value [93]. The disease progresses to progressive pulmonary hypertension and right heart failure, with death occurring within the first five years of diagnosis. The median survival is 3 years from clinical onset [86]. The differential diagnosis is with primary pulmonary hypertension, veno-occlusive disease and diffuse interstitial pulmonary fibrosis [88, 90]. Few data are available on the response to specific treatments for pulmonary arterial hypertension. A few patients have been treated with prostacyclin. No data are available on other therapeutic classes, particularly those available orally. Given the poor prognosis of pulmonary capillary haemangiomatosis and the absence of effective treatment, lung transplantation remains the treatment of choice [86, 88]. The diagnosis is confirmed by histology, which reveals a uniform proliferation of small capillaries. These form clumps that protrude into the lumens of veins and lymphatic vessels. Capillary proliferation may extend into the bronchiolar smooth muscle. Mitoses are rare. They are associated with hypertrophy of the muscular layer of the pulmonary arterioles and veins, arteriovenous intimal proliferation and focal interstitial fibrosis. Venous occlusion is considered to be reactive. Our literature review did not find any cases of pulmonary capillary haemangiomatosis treated as MAKP.

13.9. Abscesses and acute and chronic inflammatory lesions of the lung

Lung abscess is defined as a purulent, necrotic, localised process, usually more than 2 cm in diameter [66]. Abscesses are typically located in the declinal regions of the lungs, the lower lobes and the posterior segments of the upper lobes. Symptoms are non-specific and include a particularly foul-smelling productive cough, fever and chills, weight loss, chest pain, haemoptysis and dyspnoea. The chest X-ray may show a cyst with a thickened, irregular wall and blurred contours. The presence o f an aerated fluid level indicates that evacuation has occurred [66].On thoracic CT, the abscess appears as a hypodense cavity. Intravenous injection of iodinated contrast medium more clearly demarcates the hypodense centre from the raised peripheral ring. If the abscess communicates with the bronchial tree, an aerated collection forms. These cavities are generally thick-walled, but less than 5 mm, with anfractuous internal contours. They may contain multiple hydroaeric levels. Histologically, in the acute stage, the necrotic material contains numerous neutrophils. Later, the granulation tissue is replaced by collagenous tissue forming a dense fibrous capsule [3, 66]. MAKP infection can occur as early as the first days of life and pose difficult diagnostic problems with pulmonary abscess [20]. Of the 10% of MAKP diagnosed after the age of 1 year, most are due to recurrent pulmonary infections. The radiological image may then take on a cavitary appearance with a hydroaerobic level, which may point to a primary pulmonary abscess. The diagnosis is made on the basis of the multi-cystic nature of the lesion or histology. At a late stage, when the inflammatory phenomena become significant, they lead to the destruction of the cystic adenomatoid structure, making histological diagnosis difficult or even impossible [20, 95, 96, 97].

13.10. Other problems diagnosis

13.10.1. **Bronchial atresia**

It poses a differential diagnosis with MAKP type 3 where the cysts are not visible on anatomopathological examination. MRI is used t o rule out the diagnosis of MAKP [98].

13.10.2. **Neuroenteric cyst**

This is a rare anomaly corresponding to a vestigial digestive cyst located in the posterior mediastinum, with preferential lateralization to the right [99].

The echostructure is hypoechoic or frankly anechoic [100].

13.10.3. **Pleuropneumoblastoma grade I**

It poses a differential diagnosis with MAKP type 4. The distinction is often difficult because the clinical, radiological and macroscopic features are identical [101].

13.10.4. **Pneumatocele**

This is an air lesion in the lung parenchyma. Two mechanisms may be involved. It is either a lesion without its own developed wall in the immediate aftermath of the trauma due to laceration of the lung parenchyma, in which case it is a parenchymal tear, or a sequelae cavity at a distance from the trauma following a haematocele which has developed and been drained [3].

14. Hybrid malformations

The association of bronchopulmonary malformations is frequent, as shown by the classic association of an APCD and pulmonary sequestration. The association of 3 types of malformations (bronchogenic cyst, cystic adenomatoid disease and pulmonary sequestration) has also been described [25]. The hypothesis of a single bronchovascular anomaly at the origin of these abnormalities as proposed by Clements and Warner seems attractive [102]. The cause would be a lesion at the end of the bronchial tree, the aetiology of which is variable, in the form of localised trauma, ischaemia or infection. Moreover, it is not only the nature of the attack, but above all the date of onset and severity that will determine the morphological appearance of the lesion [25]. The spectrum of malformations described by Achiron et al [103] therefore tends to range from a normal lung vascularised by normal or non-normal vessels to an abnormal lung, i.e. a dysplastic lung vascularised by normal or non-normal vessels.

15. How can unnecessary lung resection be prevented?

We feel that there is little literature on this subject, and the authors do not seem to talk about their "series of failures" or "diagnostic and therapeutic errors" in MAKP. None of the authors seem to suggest a strategy for avoiding unnecessary lung resection. The clinical and radiological polymorphism of MAKP leads to diagnostic difficulties with different entities.

When faced with a unilocular cystic formation in one lobe, the problem is to gather together the arguments in favour of MAKP.

The diagnostic and therapeutic approach is based on multidisciplinary collaboration between neonatologists, paediatricians, paediatric surgeons, radiologists and experienced pathologists:

► We believe that antibiotic therapy should be continued for longer than usual, and that the disappearance of the radiological images may point towards a diagnosis of lung abscess. Elsewhere, recurrence of the radiological appearance on thoracic CT scan will tend to consolidate the diagnosis of superinfected MAKP.

► We do not insist enough on the discussion with radiologists, who will be interested in the number of cysts, the wall, the presence of a systemic vessel, etc. We must not hesitate to reconsider an established diagnosis whenever the evolution requires it. Any confrontation can only be beneficial.

▶ Intra-operative exploration must be meticulous; it is important to look for certain elements such as a systemic vessel that may have gone unnoticed on radiology, the presence of cartilage, etc.

▶ An extemporaneous anatomopathological examination did not appear to be helpful.

▶ The surgical specimen should be sent fresh and discussed with the pathologists.

CONCLUSION

MAKP is a rare malformation, most often discovered in the womb. Given its clinical and radiological polymorphism, it poses diagnostic difficulties with various entities. The differential diagnosis involves other bronchopulmonary malformations and certain acquired conditions.The diagnostic and therapeutic approach to MAKP is based on multidisciplinary collaboration: the diagnosis is based on clinical and radiological findings, and requires histological confirmation. Some diagnostic problems require discussion with experienced pathologists to avoid unnecessary lung resection.

REFERENCES

[1] **Duvergé A. Hadchouel, Lezmi G., De Blic J., Delacourt C.** Congenital lung malformations: natural history and pathogenetic hypotheses. Rev Mal Respir. **2012,** 29: 601-611.

[2] **Lezmi G., Hadchouel A., Khen-Dunlop N., Vibhushan S., Benachi A., Delacourt C.** Cystic adenomatoid malformations of the lung: diagnosis, management, pathophysiological hypotheses. Rev Pneumol Clin. **2013,** 69: 190-197.

[3] **Khalil S., Aoun N., Nedelcu C., El Rai S., Moubarak E. et al.** Cysts and cavities of the lung: semiological description and etiological approach. J Radiol. **2010,** 91: 465-473.

[4] **Bousetta K., Aloui-Kasbi N., Fitouri Z., Sammoud A., Becher S.B. et al.** Congenital lung malformations: contribution of imaging. J Pediatr Pueric. **2004,** 17: 370-379.

[5] **Margi M., Kaddouri N., Abdelhak M., Barahioui M., Benhmamouch M.** Cystic adenomatoid malformations of the lung: retrospective study of 12 observations. Rev Pneumol Clin. 2009; 65: 143-146.

[6] **Kaddour A., Chaabouni S., Meraï S., Ben Mrad S., Djilani H. et al.** Congenital cystic adenomatoid malformation of the lung. Three late-onset cases. Rev Mal Respir. **2008,** 25: 338-343.

[7] **Khemiri M., Khaldi F., Hamzaoui A., Chaouachi B., Hamzaoui M. et al.** Cystic pulmonary malformations: clinical and radiological polymorphism. About 30 observations. Rev Pneumol Clin. **2009,** 65: 333-340.

[8] **Plit M.L., Blott J.A., Lakis N., Murray J.** Clinical, radiographic and lung function features of diffuse congenital cystic adenomatoid malformation of the lung in adult. Eur Respir J. **1997,** 10: 1680-1682.

[9] **Cloutier M.M., Schaeffer D.A., Hoght D.** Congenital adenomatoid cystic disease malformation. Chest. **1993,** 103: 761-764.

[10] **Giorgio A.D., AlMansour M., Cardini C.L.** Congenital cystic adenomatoid malformation of the lung presenting as pyopneumothorax in an eighteen-year- old woman. J Thorac Cardiovasc Surg. **2001,** 122: 1034-6.

[11] **Ribet M., Pruvot F.R., Dubos J.P., Remy J., Sault M.C. et al.** Congenital cystic adenomatoid malformation of the lung. Eur J Cardio-thorac Surg. **1990,** 4: 403- 405.

[12] **Métivier A.C., Denoux Y., Tcherakian C., Puyo P., Rivaud É. et al.** Adult cystic adenomatoid pulmonary malformation: a poorly understood pathology. Rev Pneumol Clin. **2011,** 67: 275-280.

[13] **Aichaouia C., Farah S., Dabboussi S., Moatamri Z., M'hamdi S., et al.** Balloon release revealing congenital cystic adenomatoid malformation of the lung. Rev Pneumol Clin. **2012,** 68: 261-265.

[14] **Vaast P., Debarge V., Dubos J.P., Bonnevalle M., Storme L. et al.** Les malformations pulmonaires: du foetus à l'adulte, quelle prise en charge? Diagnosis and prognosis in antenatal

care. Arch Pediatr. **2004**, 11: 518-519.

[15] **Douira W., Sadfi A., Louati H., Mormech J., Ben Hassine L. et al.** Contribution of computed tomography in the diagnosis of pulmonary cystic lesions in children. J Radiol. **2008,** 89: 1621-1622.

[16] **Hourrier S., Salomon L.J., Bault J.P., Dumez Y., Ville Y.** Congenital lung malformations: antenatal diagnosis and management. Rev Mal Respir. **2011,** 28: 1017-1024.

[17] **Rittié J.L., Morelle K., Micheau P., Rancé F., Brémont F.** Medium- and long-term outcome of pulmonary malformations in children. Arch Pediatr. **2004,** 11: 520- 521.

[18] **Colombani M., Rubesova E., Potier A., Quarello E., Barth R.A. et al.** Management of fetal mediastinal deviation: a practical approach. J Radiol. **2011,** 92: 118-124.

[19] **Fourati H., Bougamra M., Ben Mansour L., Ketata H., Issa K. et al.**

Malformations bronchopulmonary in children. **2014.**

http://pe.sfrnet.org/Data/ModuleConsultationPoster/pdf/2011/1/e98a71c2-1ac9- 43a9- adc0-c421dea4cb2d.pdf.

[20] **Kieffefl F., Ferrir A., Magny J.F., Coatantiec Y., Revillon Y. et al.** Cystic adenomatoid malformation of the lung revealed in a newborn by a pulmonary abscess image. Arch Pediatr. **1996,** 3: 470-472.

[21] **Hadchouel Duvergé A., Lezmi G., De Blic J., Delacourt C.** Congenital lung malformations: natural history and pathogenic hypotheses. Rev Mal Respir. **2012,** 29: 601-611.

[22] **Wright C.** Congenital malformations of the lung. Cur Diagn Pathol. **2006,** 12: 191-201.

[23] **Pasquali R., Potier A., Gorincour G.** Fetal lung imaging. Gynecol Obstet Fer. **2008,** 36: 587-602.

[24] **Chahed J., Mekki M., Ksia A., Kechiche N., Hidouri S. et al.** Management of digestive lesions associated to congenital epidermolysis bullosa. Afr. J. Paediatr. Surg. **2015,** 12(4): 221-226.

[25] **Daudruy M., Eurin D., Ickowicz V., Liard A., Verspyck E. et al.** Contribution of ultrasound with colour and pulsed Doppler in fetal lung malformations. J Radiol. **2007,** 88: 269-276.

[26] **Salles M., Deschildre A., Bonnel C., Dubos J.P., Bonnevalle M. et al.** Diagnosis and treatment of congenital bronchopulmonary malformations: analysis o f 32 observations. Arch Pediatr. **2005,** 12: 1703-1708.

[27] **Khen N., Révillon Y.** Congenital malformations of the lung: when to operate? Rev Mal Respir. **2011,** 23: 1-9.

[28] **Dunlop N., Sarnacki S., Révillon Y.** When should congenital lung malformations be operated? Rev Pneumol Clin. **2011,** 68: 101-109.

[29] **Lejeune C., Deschildre A., Thumerelle C., Cremer R., Jaillart S. et al.** Pneumothorax revealing adenomatoid cystic malformation of the lung in a 13-year-old child.

Arch Pediatr. **1999**, 6: 863-866.

[30] **Bolca N., Topal U. ,Bayram S.** Broncho-pulmonary Sequestration: radiologic findings. Eur J Radiol. **2004**, 52: 185-191.

[31] **Wagner A., Stumbaugh A., Tigue Z., Jess E., Paquet A. et al.** Genetic analysis of congenital cystic adenomatoid malformation reveals a novel pulmonary gene: Fatty Acid Binding Protein-7. Surg Forum. **2007**, 205: S39.

[32] **Bensalem A.** Cystic bronchopulmonary malformations: anatomical, pathological and radiological aspects. Self-teaching kit. Doctoral thesis in Medicine, Faculty of Medicine of Monastir; **2009.**

[33] **Blé R., Coste K., Blanc P., Boeuf B., Lecomte B. et al.** Congenital lobar emphysema: a rare etiology of hyper-echoic lung. Gynecol Obstet Fert. **2008**, 36: 529-531.

[34] **Benachi A., Saada J., Martinovic J., De Lagausie P., Storme L. et al.** Congenital diaphragmatic hernia: antenatal care. Rev Mal Respir. **2011**, 28: 800-808.

[35] **Pennaforte T., Rakza T., Sfeir R., Aubry E., Bonnevalle M. et al.** Congenital diaphragmatic hernia: respiratory and vascular outcomes. Rev Mal Respir. **2012**, 29: 337-346.

[36] **Houssaini A., Lazguet Y., Dafiri R.** Dyspnoea at birth. Feuill Radiol. **2010**, 50: 44-47.

[37] **Chahed J., Kechiche N., Hidouri S., Aloui S., Ksia A. et al.** Neonatal Congenital Pancreatic Cyst: A Report of Three Cases. J. Preg. Child Health. **2015**, 2: 179.

[38] **Roussel A., Hascoet J.M., Desandes R., Claris O., Vieux R.** Does the regional health care organization impact the outcome of infants born with congenital diaphragmatic hernia? Arch Pediatr. **2011**, 18: 1062-1068.

[39] **Robert Y., Cuilleret, V., Vaast P., Devisme L., Mestdagh P. et al.** Prenatal thoracic MR imaging. Arch Pediatr. **2003**, 10: 340-346.

[40] **Brasseur Daudruy M., Ickowicz V., Eurin D.** Fetal MRI: indications, limits and dangers. Gynecol Obst et Fert. **2007**, 35: 678-683.

[41] **Storme L., Pennaforte T., Rakza T., Fily A., Sfeir R. et al.** Intra- and post-natal medical management of congenital hernia of the diaphragm. Arch Pediatr. **2010**, 17: S85-S92.

[42] **Coste C., Jouvencel P., Debuch C., Argote C., Lavrand F. et al.** Late-onset congenital diaphragmatic hernias: diagnostic difficulties. A propos de deux cas. Arch Pediatr. **2004**, 11: 929-931.

[43] **Jellali M.A., Ben Salem R., Zrig A., Saad J., Mnari W. et al.** Late-onset congenital diaphragmatic hernias in children. À propos de 32 cases. **2014.**

http://pe.sfrnet.org/Data/ModuleConsultationPoster/pdf/2010/1/2b078785-dfff-4b68-8937-1f118050f0ba.pdf.

[44] **Dubois A., Storme L., Jaillardz S., Truffert P., Rio Y. et al.** Les hernies congénitales des coupoles diaphragmatiques: étude rétrospective de 123 observations recueillies dans le service de médecine néonatale du CHRU de Lille entre 1985 et 1996. Arch Pediatr. **2000**, 7: 132-142.

[45] **Aloui-kasbi N., Bellagha I., Hammou A.** Pulmonary sequestration: particular clinical

and radiological features. Arch Pediatr. **2004,** 11: 394-396.

[46] **Kabiri H., Smahi M., Achir A., Herrak L., Alaziz S. et al.** Pulmonary sequestration. A propos de 5 cas. Med Maghr. **2000,** 83: 7-12.

[47] **Michel M., Isart D.** Pulmonary sequestration. Press Med. **2004,** 33: 794.

[48] **Carette M.F., Frey I., Tassart M., Lebreton C., Khalilber A.** Imagerie des séquestrations. Feuill Radiol. **2002,** 42: 384-390.

[49] **Michaux H., Noel J.B., Besnard M., Prevot M., Sauvage P.J.** Extra-lobar sequestration associated with a bronchogenic cyst. A case report. J Radiol. **2010,** 91: 1164-1167.

[50] **Ko S.F., Ng S.H., Lee T.Y., Wang Y.L., Liang C.D. et al.** Non-invasive imaging of broncho-pulmonary sequestration. Am J Roentgenol. **2000,** 175: 1005-1012.

[51] **Kabiri E.H., Atoini F., Jidal M., Rguibi M., Alaoui T.** Sequestration of the postero-basal segment of the right lower pulmonary lobe. Ann chir. **2006,** 131: 547-549.

[52] **Bachmeyer C., Lavoléb A., Assouad J., Khalil A.** An asymptomatic lung mass. Rev Med Intern. **2009,** 30: 438-439.

[53] **Pefoubou Y., Galloy M.A., Mainard L., Pecastaings M., Antunes L. et al.** Pulmonary sequestrations: contribution of new imaging techniques in the foetus and neonate. Feuill Radiol. **2005,** 45: 97-106.

[54] **Babu R., Kyle P., Spicer R.D.** Prenatal sonographic features of congenital lobar emphysema. Fetal Diagn Ther. **2001,** 16: 200-202.

[55] **Quinton A.E, Smoleniec J.S.** Congenital lobar emphysema - the disappearing chest mass: antenatal ultrasound appearence. Ultrasound Obstet Gynecol. **2001,** 17: 169- 171.

[56] **Thakral C.L., Maji D.C., Sajwani M.J.** Congenital lobar emphysema: experience with 21 cases. Pediatr Surg Int. **2001,** 17: 88-91.

[57] **Salem R., Ben Salem A., Jellali M.A., Zrig A., Njim L. et al.** Giant lobar emphysema versus emphysema compensatory emphysema. **2014.** http://pe.sfrnet.org/Data/ModuleConsultationPoster/pdf/2009/1/ca5104e1-c2a4-4129- 9a99-e602fbc00b0a.pdf.

[58] **Karnack I., Senocak M.E., Ciftci A.O.** Congenital lobar emphysema: diagnostic and therapeutic considerations. J Pediatr Surg. **1999,** 34: 1347-1351.

[59] **Adzick S., Harrison M.R., Crombleholme T.M., Flake A.W., Howell L.J.** Fetal lung lesions: management and outcome. Am J Obstet Gynecol. **1998,** 179: 884-889.

[60] **Shanmugam G., MacArthur K., Pollock J.C.** Congenital lung malformations: antenatal and post-natal evaluation and management. Eur J Cardiothorac Surg. **2005,** 27: 45-52.

[61] **Bogers A.J., Hazebroek F.W., Molenaar J.** Surgical treatment of congenital bronchopulmonary disease in children. Europ J Cardiothorac Surg. **1993,** 7: 117-119.

[62] **Lefevre C., Marsa A., Doana C., Liesseb A., Bonnevalle M. et al.** Asthma belatedly revealing a bronchogenic cyst. Arch Pediatr. **2011,** 18: 1336-1338.

[63]   Barthesa F., Cazesb A., Bagana P., Badiaa A., Vlasa C. et al. Mediastinal cysts: diagnostic approach and treatment. Rev Pneumol Clin. **2010**, 66: 52- 62.

[64]   McAdams H.P., Kirejczyk W.M., Rosado-de-Christenson M.L., Matsumoto S. Bronchogenic cyst: imaging features with clinical and histo-pathologic correlation. Radiol. **2000**, 217: 441-446.

[65]   Yoon Y.C., Lee K.S., Kim T.S., Kim J., Shim Y.M. et al. Intra-pulmonary bronchogenic cyst: CT and pathologic findings in five adult patients. Am J Roentgenol. **2002**, 179: 167-170.

[66] Grosse C., Bankier A.A., Remmelink M., Gevenois P.A. Diagnosis of hyperclartes and cystic pulmonary images in adults. EMC Pneumology. **2007**, 6-090-C-50.

[67] Aktogu S., Yuncu G., Halilcolar H., Ermete S., Buduneli T. Bronchogenic cysts: clinicopathological presentation and treatment. Eur Respir J. **1996**, 9: 2017-2021.

[68] Belcher E., Abbasi M.A., Hansell D.M., Folkes L., Nicholson A.G. et al. Persistent interstitial pulmonary emphysema requiring pneumonectomy. J Thoracic Cardiovasc Surg. **2009**, 138: 237-239.

[69] Gourrier E., Phan F., Wood C., Mokhtari M., Chenel C. Interest and limitations of selective bronchial obstruction in neonatal unilateral interstitial emphysema. Arch Pediatr. **1997**, 4: 751-754.

[70] Macklin M.T. Malignant interstitial emphysema of the lungs and mediastinum as an important occult complication in many respiratory diseases and other conditions: an interpretation of clinical literature in the light of laboratory experiment. Med. **1944**, 23: 281-358.

[71] Freysdottir D., Olutoye O., Langston C., Fernandes C.J., Tatevian N. Spontaneous pulmonary interstitial emphysema in a term unventilated infant. Pediatr Pulmonol. **2006**, 41: 374-378.

[72] Jassal M.S., Benson J.E., Peter J., Mogayzel P.J. Spontaneous resolution of diffuse persistent pulmonary interstitial emphysema. Pediatr Pulmonol. **2008**, 43: 615-619.

[73] Rao J., Hochman M.I., Miller G. Localized persistent pulmonary interstitial emphysema. J Pediatr Surg. **2006**, 41: 1191- 1193.

[74] Matta R., Matta J., Hage P., Nassif Y., Mansour N. et al. Diffuse Persistent Interstitial Pulmonary Emphysema treated by lobectomy. Ann Thoracic Surg. **2011**, 92: e73-75.

[75] Corsini I., Pratesi S., Dani C. Pulmonary interstitial emphysema after resolution of relapsing pneumothorax and discontinuation of mechanical ventilation.An atypical case in a preterm infant. J Matern Fetal Neonat Med. **2013**, 16: 1-4.

[76] Gonçalves C.A., Martin V., Ochoa A., Carvalho P. Pulmonary lobar interstitial emphysema. Fetal Pediatr Pathol. **2009**, 28: 192-197.

[77] Deschildre S. Diagnosis, aetiologies and evolution of bronchiectasis in children. Rev Pneumol. **2001**, 57: 1-13.

[78] Barker A.F. Bronchiectasis. N Engl J Med. **2002**, 346: 1383-1393.

[79] **Nouira K.** Dilation of the bronchi and emphysema. **2014.**
http://www.medecinesfax.org/fra/search/p/4/Dilatation%20des%20bronches%20
and%20emphys%C3%A8me%20Nouira.

[80] **Guerrouj H., Mouaden A., Ghfir I., Ben Rais N.** Intérêt de la scintigraphie pulmonaire de perfusion dans les dilatations des bronches de l'enfant. Med Nucl. **2013,** 37: 429-431.

[81] **Kalendarov D., Hubert D.** Management of bronchiectasis without antibiotic therapy. Rev Pneumol Clin. **2001,** 57: 1S31-1S36.

[82] **Stocker J.T.** Post-infarction peripheral cysts of the lung. Pediatr Pathol. **1987,** 7: 111-117.

[83] **Lytrivi I., Reingold S., Ramaswamy P.** Neonatal left pulmonary artery occlusion and post-infarction cysts of the left lung: cause and effect? Pediatr Cardiol. **2008,** 29: 1002-1003.

[84] **Stocker J.T., McGill L.C., Orsini E.N.** Post-infarction peripheral cysts of the lung in pediatric patients: a possible cause of idiopathic spontaneous pneumothorax. Pediatr Pulmonol. **1985,** 1: 7-18.

[85] **Marchac V., Chigot V., Courtel J.V., Brunelle F.** Pulmonary vascular malformations in children. EMC Pediatr. **2001,** 32- 330- A-30.

[86] **Montani D., Dorfmuller P., Maitre S., Jaïs X., Sitbon O. et al.** Veno-occlusive disease and pulmonary capillary haemangiomatosis. Press Med. **2010,** 39: 134-143.

[87] **Havlik D.M., Massie L.W., Williams W.L., Crooks L.A.** Pulmonary capillary hemangiomatosis like foci. Am J Clin Pathol. **2000,** 113: 655-666.

[88] **Oviedo A., Abramson L.P., Worthington R., Dainauskas J.R., Crawford S.E. Congenitalpulmonary capillary hemangiomatosis: report of two cases and review of the Literature. Pediatr Pulmonol. 2003, 36: 253-256.**

[89] **Almagro P., Julia J., Sanjaume M., González G., Casalots J. et al.** Pulmonary capillary hemangiomatosis associated with primary pulmonary hypertension: report of 2 new cases and review of 35 cases from the literature. Medecine. **2002,** 81: 417-424.

[90] **Langleben D., Heneghan J.H., Batten A.P., Wang N., Fitch N. et al.** Familial pulmonary capillary hemangiomatosis resulting in primary hypertension. Ann Intern Med. **1988,** 109: 106-109.

[91] **Al Fawaz I.M., Al Mobaireek K.F., Al Suhaibani M., Ashour M.** Pulmonary capillary hemangiomatosis: a case report and review of literature. Pediatr Pulmonol. **1995,** 19: 243-248.

[92] **Lippert J.L., White C.S., Cameron E.W., Sun C.C., Liang X. et al.** Pulmonary capillary hemangiomatosis: radiographic appearance. J Thorac Imaging. **1998,** 13: 49-51.

[93] **Grando A.** A case of pulmonary capillary haemangiomatosis in an infant of

11 months. **2014.** http://www.despedara.org/cours-des/mem-20080000-hemangiomatose-capillary-pulmonary-infant.pdf.

[94] **Dufour B., Maitre S., Humbert M., Capron F., Simonneau G. et al.** High- resolution CT of the chest in four patients with pulmonary capillary hemangiomatosis or pulmonary

veno-oclussive disease. Am J Roentgenol. **1998,** 171: 1321-1324.

[95] Dahabreha J., Zisis Ch., Vassiliou M., Arnogiannaki N. Congenital cystic adenomatoid malformation in an adult presenting as lung abscess. Eur J Cardio-thorac Surg. **2000,** 18: 720-723.

[96] Pelizzo G., Barbi E., Codricha D., Lemboa M., Zennaro F. et al. Chronic inflammation in congenital cystic adenomatoid malformation: an underestimated risk factor? J Pediatr Surg. **2009,** 44: 616-619.

[97] Huang H., Talbot A., Liu K., Chen C., Fang H. Infected cystic adenomatoid malformation in an adult. Ann Thorac Surg. **2004,** 78: 337-339.

[98] Nouri A., Ksia A., Bouzaffara B., Munsterer O., Hidouri S. et al. A new operative **approach for long-gap esophageal atresia. J. Indian Assoc. Pediatr. Surg. 2019, 24: 132-134.**

[99] Ballouhey Q., Brémont F., Rittié J.L., Baunin C., Danjoux M. et al. Pulmonary sequestration and enteric cyst: 2 expressions of the same abnormality. Arch Pediatr. **2012,** 19: 27-30.

[100] Morris M., Lim F., Livingston C., Polzin J., Crombleholme M. High-risk fetal congenital pulmonary airway malformations have a variable response to steroids. J Pediatr Surg. **2009,** 44: 60-65.

[101] Lopez-Andreu J.A., Ferris-Tortajada J., Gomez J. Pleuro-pulmonary blastoma and congenital cystic malformations. J Pediatr. **1996,** 129: 773-774.

[102] Clements B.S, Warner J.O. Pulmonary sequestration and related congenital bronchopulmonary vascular malformations: nomenclature and classification based on anatomical and embryological considerations. Thorax. **1987,** 42: 401- 408.

[103] Achiron R., Hegesh J., Yagel S. Fetal lung lesions: a spectrum of diseases. New classification based on pathogenesis, two-dimensional and Color Doppler ultrasound. Ultrasound Obstet Gynecol. **2004,** 24: 107-114.

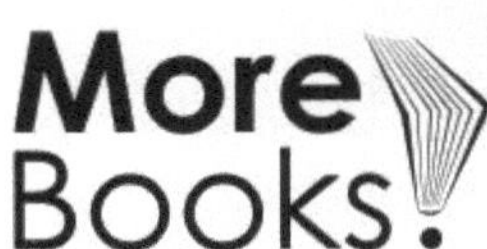

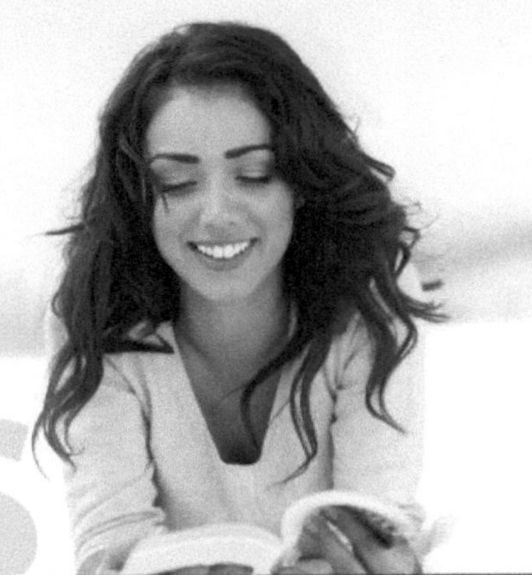

Buy your books fast and straightforward online - at one of world's fastest growing online book stores! Environmentally sound due to Print-on-Demand technologies.

Buy your books online at
www.morebooks.shop

Kaufen Sie Ihre Bücher schnell und unkompliziert online – auf einer der am schnellsten wachsenden Buchhandelsplattformen weltweit! Dank Print-On-Demand umwelt- und ressourcenschonend produziert.

Bücher schneller online kaufen
www.morebooks.shop

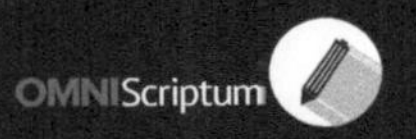

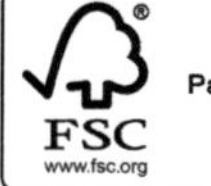

Printed by Books on Demand GmbH, Norderstedt / Germany